Clinical Teaching & Evaluation Manual for
Respiratory Care

California College for Health Sciences
222 West 24th Street
National City, CA 91950

Acknowledgments: Special thanks to Diane Kizer, Edward Moser, Lori Wiedner, Terry Marshall, Mark Vinzant, Joy Tapscott, Michael Johnson, and Michael Cronin for their help and cooperation in formatting, reviewing and editing this edition of the manual.

Published by:

California College for Health Sciences

222 West 24th Street

National City, CA 91950

PREFACE

The *Clinical Teaching & Evaluation Manual for Respiratory Care* was developed for use in the evaluation of students who enroll in the advanced standing respiratory care programs offered by California College for Health Sciences (CCHS). It is used by CCHS to diagnose the clinical deficiencies of students at the time of entry into the program. It is used again to determine the clinical proficiency of the students at the time of program completion. In addition, the students are encouraged to use the manual to assist them in eliminating any diagnosed deficiencies prior to the final clinical evaluation.

The clinical manual consists of a series of self-instructional modules that can be used for both laboratory and clinical training. In the laboratory setting, the modules provide an introduction to the equipment used and to the steps followed in the performance of basic respiratory care procedures. For clinical training, the manual provides step-by-step procedures for the therapeutic modalities that are commonly performed at entrance into the practice of respiratory therapy.

The manual was designed to facilitate the development of clinical proficiency in the delivery of respiratory care. It was intended to serve the dual role of an instructional manual for respiratory therapy students and an evaluation manual for respiratory therapy educators. By providing these two components in a single manual, similar performance expectations are communicated to both students and evaluators.

An additional use for the manual is the evaluation of the clinical proficiency of practicing respiratory care personnel. The evaluation procedures can be incorporated into an annual performance review used to assess and diagnose the clinical functioning of employees. If deficiencies are found, the manual can also be used to assist in the remediation of employee weaknesses.

The authors are aware of the local and regional variations in the procedures used for the delivery of respiratory care. For this reason, an effort was made to identify the procedures that are most commonly performed and to present them in the manner that appears to be most widely accepted in this country. As the procedures used in respiratory care become more standardized across the nation, the manual will be updated to reflect the changes that take place.

The first edition of the clinical manual was written in 1982 by Darol L. Graham, PhD and Jan Y. Guynes, PhD, RRT. Procedures used for oxygen therapy and ventilatory assistance for infants were added by Diane Kizer, RRT and Edward Moser, RRT for the second edition (1984). The third edition contains a number of revisions and additions that have been incorporated into the earlier editions by Darol L. Graham, PhD and Diane Kizer, RRT.

Table of Contents

Section One: Support Skills

Section Two: Ancillary Procedures

Table of Contents (continued)

Section Three: Clinical Procedures

Table of Contents (continued)

Section Four: Evaluation Procedures

Proficiency Evaluation Process
    Evaluation Procedures
    Data Recording Procedures
    Proficiency Evaluation Forms
    Appendix

INTRODUCTION

The development of clinical competence is a major objective of respiratory care education. This manual was prepared to assist respiratory therapy students in their efforts to develop such competence. To facilitate the attainment of this objective, the manual provides detailed guidelines for learning the most commonly performed respiratory care procedures.

The clinic provides the setting in which the respiratory care practitioner can demonstrate the ability to integrate and apply the theoretical concepts acquired in the classroom. The quality of patient care provided by the beginning practitioner is a reflection of the type and quality of clinical training that the practitioner received as a student.

The manual is divided into three major sections designated as: **Support Skills**, **Ancillary Procedures**, and **Clinical Procedures**. Each section is further divided into a series of modules that organize commonly performed skills and procedures into related units. Each module of the manual consists of an instructional component and an evaluation component.

The purpose of the instructional components is to supplement the didactic portion of respiratory therapy training programs. Each of the components includes: (1) a brief introduction; (2) a list of module objectives; (3) a learning resource including indications, contraindications, and hazards for the procedure; and (4) instructions for performing each procedure.

The learning resources contained in the modules provide a brief review of the essential content related to each of the procedures to be performed. Following the review of relevant content, highly detailed directions for performing the respiratory care procedures are provided. The directions are intended to be sufficiently clear and distinct that they could be followed by someone who is unfamiliar with the procedures.

The purpose of the evaluation components of the manual is to measure student performance in either a laboratory or clinical setting. Educators can use the instruments for student diagnosis and placement or for final evaluation of clinical competence. In addition, the instruments can be used by students when learning to perform the skills and procedures or to evaluate peers during evaluation practice sessions. Because of the versatility and level of detail of the instruments, they have been found equally useful for both training and evaluation.

Organization of the Manual

It was previously indicated that the manual is organized into three major sections. The following discussion provides a brief description of the contents of the three sections and a rationale for their organization and format.

Support Skills

The first section contains a collection of clinical skills that make up an integral part of many respiratory care procedures. The *Support Skills* are organized into four major groups entitled: **Infection Control, Basic Patient Assessment, Data Management,** and **Communication Skills.** Some of the skills, such as *Maintaining Asepsis* and *Reporting Observations*, appear as component steps in virtually all procedures and are seldom performed except as steps in one of the procedures.

The primary reason for creating a separate section for the *Support Skills* was to minimize redundancy in **Sections II** and **III** of the manual. Such redundancy would occur whenever one of the skills appeared as a performance step in one of the clinical or ancillary procedures. Placement of the *Support Skills* in a separate section with unique identifiers, permits referencing of one of the skills whenever it appears as a step in one of the procedures. If a detailed description of one of these procedural steps is needed at the time it is being performed or evaluated, the user can simply turn back to **Section I** for the description.

Ancillary Procedures

The term *Ancillary Procedure* is used to identify any of the respiratory care procedures that is frequently performed without a specific order from the physician. Such procedures are usually performed whenever the need arises during the administration of other therapy. For example, *Ancillary Procedures* such as *Tracheal Suctioning* and *Arterial Blood Sampling* are ordinarily performed in conjunction with the administration of *Continuous Mechanical Ventilation*. Although the *Ancillary Procedures* occasionally appear on a physician's order, they are most likely to be performed during the administration of another procedure.

Clinical Procedures

The term *Clinical Procedure* was reserved for those respiratory therapy procedures that ordinarily require a physician's order for implementation. The *clinical procedures,* **presented in the third section of the manual,** encompass the major therapeutic modalities used in respiratory care. The ability to perform these procedures in a competent manner requires prior mastery of virtually all of the *Support Skills* and *Ancillary Procedures*.

Performance Definitions

The evaluation component of the manual consists of two parts, the *performance definitions* and the *proficiency evaluation forms*. The performance definitions provide detailed specifications of the characteristics of correct performance. The definitions used to evaluate the clinical and ancillary procedures are organized into three components: **Performance Steps**, **Essential Tasks**, and **Evaluation Criteria**. The purpose and use of each of the components should be understood before attempting to use them.

Performance Steps

Each procedure is broken down into a series of major steps that are performed in sequence. The steps are listed in the first column of the performance definition tables in their order of performance. The steps provide an organizational scheme for the evaluation instruments and for the major components to be evaluated.

Essential Tasks

The essential tasks provide a further breakdown of each procedural step. The tasks are listed in the second column of the performance definition tables, adjacent to the respective performance steps. In order for a particular step to be completed, each associated task must be performed.

Evaluation Criteria

The evaluation criteria found in the third column of the performance definition tables provide the standards of acceptable performance for each of the essential tasks. These criteria enable the evaluator to determine whether or not the tasks are performed correctly. Each criterion is an observable behavior that can be assessed objectively during evaluation.

It should be noted that, occasionally, an evaluation criterion is simply indicated by the letters **SOP**. The letters refer to a *standard operating procedure* such as the assembly or testing of a particular piece of equipment according to the manufacturer's equipment manual. **SOP** is also used to define criteria that are determined by hospital protocol. For clarification of some particular **SOP**, it may be necessary to consult the appropriate equipment or procedure manual.

It was suggested earlier that certain performance steps are common to several procedures. These steps were defined as support skills and presented as a separate section of evaluation instruments. Whenever one of the support skills appears as a performance step in a clinical or ancillary procedure, the *Essential Tasks* and *Evaluation Criteria* columns contain the word "See" followed by the letters *SSE* and the number of the appropriate support skill. This code identifies a particular *Support Skill Evaluation*. Whenever such a code is encountered during the evaluation of a procedure, it is necessary to turn back to **Section I** for a description of the *Essential Tasks* and *Evaluation Criteria* for the skill.

Proficiency Evaluation Forms

The *Proficiency Evaluation Forms* are located at the back of this manual. The forms are used for recording the results obtained during clinical evaluation sessions. A separate form is provided for each procedure to be evaluated. The *Proficiency Evaluation Forms* provide space for recording: *Pertinent identification information, evaluation results for each performance step, and evaluator comments pertaining to either a particular step in the procedure or to the procedure as a whole.*

When using the *Proficiency Evaluation Forms*, performance on each step is recorded as either *Acceptable (A)*, *Unacceptable (U)*, or *Not evaluated (N)*. To be considered *Acceptable*, all *Essential Tasks* must be performed and they must be performed in the manner specified by the *Evaluation Criteria*. This means that *perfection* is expected in the performance of each procedural step. Experience indicates that mastery performance is an entirely realistic expectation. In most instances, students who know precisely what is expected of them and who have sufficient opportunity to practice are able to perform the procedures without error.

It should be pointed out that the performance of certain *Essential Tasks*, and even some entire *Performance Steps, cannot be observed* visually. For example, it may be impossible for the evaluator to determine what is transpiring during *Chart Review* except through discussion. For this reason, the student should verbalize his or her thoughts at such times and should be prepared to answer questions posed by the evaluator. Proper discretion should be used whenever such conversations are conducted in the patient's room.

A final comment should be made regarding local and regional variations in the performance of respiratory care procedures. Although we have tried to present the generally preferred methods of performing the procedures, there may be alternative methods that are equally acceptable. The most common variation is in the sequence of performing the component tasks of certain procedural steps. In arbitrary situations, such as the performance of certain tasks, decisions are most appropriately made at the local level. These and any other procedural variations should be identified by the instructor or evaluator, noted in the manual, and communicated to the student or employee.

The clinical manual is considered appropriate for the training and evaluation of *both respiratory therapists and respiratory therapy technicians*. Although the two types of practitioners may function with differing levels of supervision, both are expected to be able to demonstrate proficiency in the performance of a common set of basic clinical procedures. Since the steps that are followed in performing a particular respiratory therapy procedure are essentially the same regardless of the level of practice, the evaluation instruments provided in this manual should be appropriate across the entire range.

Section One
Support Skills

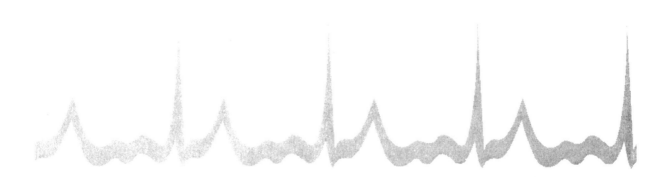

Module 1.0

Infection Control

A major concern in all hospitals is controlling the spread of infection from patient to patient, employee to patient, or patient to employee. Special precautions must be taken to prevent the transmission of pathogenic organisms to any individual who may be susceptible to infection by the organism. Hospital employees are responsible for performing their duties in a manner that helps in controlling the spread of infection.

Objectives

Upon completion of this module, you will be able to:

1. Discuss the procedures used to implement the OSHA regulations for universal precautions.

2. Describe the importance of maintaining asepsis while performing routine patient care.

3. Perform proper handwashing technique.

4. Define and differentiate between different procedures used for patient isolation.

5. Perform proper isolation technique.

6. Thoroughly clean respiratory therapy equipment in preparation for disinfection or sterilization procedures.

The rapidly increasing number of patients who are infected with the Hepatitis B virus (HBV) or the Human Immunodeficiency Virus (HIV) has resulted in a growing concern about infection control issues. In an effort to reduce exposure to the HBV and HIV viruses, the Occupational Safety and Hazards Administration (OSHA) has taken steps to regulate the procedures followed in the operation of healthcare institutions.

OSHA regulations are written to protect employees and patients from exposing susceptible areas of parenteral tissue, mucus membrane and nonintact skin to blood-borne pathogens. According to the regulations, the key to infection control involves the use of "Universal Precautions". This term refers to an infection control system which assumes that every direct contact with bodily fluids is infectious and that every employee who may be in contact with bodily fluids must be protected as if the fluids were infected with HBV or HIV. (See appendix for copy of "Universal Precautions" and the 1991 updated recommendations for preventing transmission of HIV and HBV to patients during exposure-prone invasive procedures.)

Bodily fluids are defined by the Centers for Disease Control (CDC) as those fluids that are linked directly to the transmission of HIV or HBV. Such fluids include: blood, blood products, semen, vaginal secretions, cerebrospinal fluid, synovial fluid, pleural fluid, peritoneal fluid, pericardial fluid, amniotic fluid, and any solution which could contain HBV or HIV viruses.

OSHA requires that all hospital employees comply with the regulations covering the use of universal precautions whenever the employee is at risk of coming in contact with bodily fluids. Such precautions are required whether the patient is known to be infected with HBV or HIV or not. Universal precautions are necessary because of the limitations of HIV testing and because of the need to protect patient confidentiality.

Infection control procedures require strict adherence to universal precautions. They also include maintaining asepsis and following prescribed isolation procedures while performing routine patient care. This module addresses the procedures used to protect both patients and hospital employees from the risk of infection.

Support Skill 1.1
Handwashing Technique

One of the important ways that hospital employees can reduce the risk of patient infection is by maintaining proper personal hygiene. Of particular importance is the attention given to handwashing by employees who perform patient care activities. The hands should be thoroughly scrubbed and rinsed before and after administering patient care or handling equipment used for patient care. In addition, handwashing should be performed anytime during patient care that contamination of the hands is suspected, thus posing a risk to the patient or yourself.

It is not possible to remove all microorganisms from the hands by washing. The effectiveness of handwashing can be optimized, however, by performing the procedure properly. Before washing the hands, all jewelry and garments should be removed from the hands and wrists. If a wristwatch is worn, it should be moved above the wrist and remain there until the patient care procedure is completed. Important considerations during handwashing include vigorous scrubbing for at least two minutes with disinfectant soap. All surfaces of the hands and wrists (3 to 4 inches above the hands), including the areas between the fingers and under and around all nail surfaces, should receive attention. Following thorough rinsing, techniques that avoid recontaminating the washed area should be employed when turning off the water and drying the skin.

Procedure for Handwashing

The following steps are recommended for washing hands:

1. Remove all jewelry from your hands and wrists. If you are wearing a watch, move it above your wrist.

2. Turn on the water and let it run continuously throughout the procedure.

3. Wet your hands and apply soap.

4. Thoroughly scrub (for two minutes) all surfaces of the hands and wrists, including:

   • Palms and backs of hands.
   • Fingers and surfaces between, under and around all nail surfaces.
   • Wrists (3 to 4 inches above the hands).

5. Rinse your hands thoroughly under running water from wrists to fingers.

6. Dry your hands and wrists thoroughly with a clean towel.

7. Turn off the faucet with the towel used to dry the hands.

Support Skill 1.2
Maintaining Asepsis

It is essential that aseptic technique be used by employees while performing all patient care activities that could possibly result in infection of the patient. In applying aseptic technique, handwashing is one of the most important and most frequently performed activities. Diligence in handwashing is of no avail, however, unless equal attention is given to other means of maintaining asepsis. Only sterile or disinfected equipment, supplies and medications should be used. When using these items, they should always be handled with good aseptic technique. If contamination occurs for any reason, these items should be replaced and the hands rewashed. If in doubt regarding the status of equipment or supplies, contamination should be assumed and they should not be used.

Procedure for Maintaining Asepsis

When performing respiratory therapy procedures, universal precautions should be followed and asepsis should be maintained at all times. The following specific steps for maintaining asepsis are recommended:

1. Wash your hands before and after performing all respiratory care procedures in the manner presented in **SSE 1.1**.

2. Take universal precautions whenever the possibility of exposure to body fluids exists by wearing:

   - Gloves
   - Mask
   - Eye protection

3. Obtain only sterile or disinfected equipment, medications and supplies.

4. When handling all equipment, medications and supplies, avoid contact with possible contaminants.

5. Replace any item that you suspect has become contaminated.

6. Repeat handwashing following any contact with possible contaminants.

Support Skill 1.3
Isolation Technique

Certain hospital situations require special precautions to avoid the spread of infection. Whenever there is a serious risk of transferring an infection from one individual to another, isolation techniques are necessary.

Isolation may be implemented to prevent a patient from transmitting a highly communicable disease or to protect a patient who has reduced resistance to infection. This latter situation, known as *protective* or *reverse isolation*, is commonly employed with burn victims and patients with impaired resistance due to chemotherapy or other factors that reduce the effectiveness of the body's natural immune processes.

Special isolation rooms or, if isolation is not possible, private rooms should be used for isolation. All persons entering an isolation room should wear appropriate protective clothing. Such clothing may include a gown, gloves, mask, hair covering and shoe coverings. If possible, only disposable equipment and supplies should be used with patients with highly contagious diseases. Nondisposable items removed from an isolation room should be bagged before leaving the room and placed in a second protective bag immediately outside the room. All supplies and equipment used with patients in isolation should be kept separate from noncontaminated items until after cleaning and sterilization.

Prior to use, protective clothing should be stored in an anteroom or suitable storage area directly outside the isolation room. Protective attire should be put on and removed in a manner that minimizes risk of contamination. The sequence and associated rationale for putting on isolation attire for protecting a patient from potential infection are provided in **Table 1-1** on the following page.

DRESSING FOR ISOLATION SITUATIONS

ITEM SEQUENCE	RATIONALE
1. Hair Covering	In case the mask needs to be replaced during the procedure, it can be accomplished without first removing the hair covering.
2. Mask	The mask should be placed over the mouth and nose as soon as possible to prevent aerosol droplets from contaminating other articles of attire. (If there is little likelihood that it will be necessary to replace the mask during the procedure, it should be put on before the hair covering.)
3. Eye Covering	Goggles or eye protection should be placed over the eyes to prevent exposure of the mucus membranes of the eye to bodily fluids.
4. Shoe Coverings	The shoes are covered before putting on the gown to prevent possible contamination of the gown through contact with the floor while covering the shoes.
5. Gown	The gown is put on before the gloves because the gloves might become contaminated while tying the gown.
6. Gloves	By slipping the gloves on last, they are most likely to remain free from contamination.

Table 1-1.

The sequence in **Table 1-1** is less critical when the purpose of isolation is to protect you from patient contamination. Nevertheless, it is recommended that the same procedure be followed at all times. By adopting a standard sequence, you will develop habits that always assure proper patient protection.

REMOVING ISOLATION ATTIRE

ITEM SEQUENCE	RATIONALE
1. Shoe Coverings	If care is used, shoe coverings can be removed with contaminated gloves without contaminating yourself or your personal attire.
2. Gloves	It is difficult to remove the gown or mask with gloved hands without contaminating your body or clothing.
3. Gown	The gown is removed next because the mask should remain in place as long as possible to avoid inhaling airborne pathogens.
4. Mask	If the hair covering is under the mask, the mask must be removed first.
5. Eye Covering	If the hair covering is under the eye covering, the eye covering must be removed first.
6. Hair Covering	If the mask is put on first, the order of removing the mask and hair covering is reversed.

Table 1-2.

The recommended sequence for removing isolation attire is provided in ***Table 1-2***. The accompanying rationale is designed to protect you from contamination during the removal process. The sequence for removing protective attire is not critical when the patient is in reverse isolation. It is recommended, however, that you develop the habit of removing isolation attire in the same sequence at all times.

Protective attire should always be removed immediately prior to leaving an isolation room in which a highly contagious patient is confined. When the patient is in reverse isolation, it is preferable to remove the clothing immediately outside the room. Protective garments should never be reused without cleaning and should be placed in an appropriate container for cleaning (if reusable) or disposal.

Procedure for Maintaining Isolation

When administering care to a patient in isolation, follow universal precautions and dress in the necessary protective clothing according to the following procedure:

1. Wash your hands according to the procedure described in **SSE 1.1**.

2. If the isolation category requires a hair covering, place the covering over your hair ensuring complete coverage.

3. If the isolation category requires a mask, thoroughly cover your mouth and nose with a mask.

4. If the isolation category requires eye protection, place the covering over the eyes ensuring complete coverage.

5. If the isolation category requires shoe coverings, place the coverings over your shoes ensuring complete coverage.

6. Put on the gown according to the following procedure:

    • Pick up the gown by grasping the back of the neck. (Avoid touching the front of the gown.)
    • Place your hands inside the sleeves. (Avoid touching the cuff or front of the gown.)
    • Fasten the ties at the neck.
    • Close the gown in back and fasten the waist tie.

7. If the isolation category requires gloves, select the appropriate size and type of gloves (sterile or "clean") and put on the gloves ensuring complete coverage of the hands and wrists.

8. Upon entering the room, empty all contaminated liquids and place disposable equipment into the proper receptacles.

9. Place all contaminated, nondisposable equipment in a bag and seal it. The bagged equipment should be placed inside a clean bag (held by a second person outside the isolation room). The second bag should be sealed and appropriately labeled as isolation equipment.

10. Remove the shoe coverings and discard in the appropriate receptacle.

11. Remove the gloves and discard in the appropriate receptacle.

12. Remove the gown according to the following procedure:

    - Unfasten the waist and neck ties.
    - Pull off one sleeve by reaching under the cuff.
    - Using the sleeve-covered hand, pull off the second sleeve.
    - Fold the gown inside out.
    - Discard in the appropriate receptacle.

13. Remove the mask and discard in the appropriate receptacle.

14. Remove the hair covering and discard in the appropriate receptacle.

15. After leaving the room, wash your hands according to the procedure described in **SSE 1.1.**

Support Skill 1.4
Cleaning Equipment

The first step in the decontamination of respiratory therapy equipment is thorough washing to remove secretions, blood, and other substances that may adhere to the surface. This equipment may be washed either manually or with an automatic machine. Regardless of the method used for cleaning equipment, it should be rinsed thoroughly to remove soap, detergent or loosened debris. During the entire process, universal precautions must be observed.

Procedure for Cleaning Equipment

Prior to disinfection or sterilization, it is recommended that all equipment be cleaned according to the following procedure:

1. Take universal precautions to avoid contact with equipment or supplies that may be contaminated with body fluids by wearing protective:

    • Gloves
    • Mask
    • Eye covering

2. Prepare equipment to be disinfected or sterilized in the following manner:

    • Discard disposable equipment and supplies.
    • Dispose of equipment contaminated with body fluids in a hazardous waste receptacle.
    • Disassemble equipment down to its smallest components.

3. Wash immersible items in hot detergent solution, scrubbing to remove debris.

4. Rinse the equipment thoroughly to remove all traces of soap.

5. If the equipment is to be sterilized, thoroughly dry it with a clean towel, heat lamp or drying cabinet.

Evaluation of Infection Control Support Skills

The following definitions are provided for use whenever the respective Infection Control Support Skills are evaluated during the performance of a Clinical or Ancillary Procedure. In order for performance of the skills to be considered acceptable, all Essential Tasks are to be performed according to the accompanying Evaluation Criteria. Any deviation from the following task sequence or criteria must be approved by the evaluator.

SSE 1.1 Handwashing Technique		
Performance	**Essential Tasks**	**Evaluation Criteria**
A. Wash Hands	1. Prepares hands and wrists	a. All jewelry removed b. Watch moved above the wrist c. Uncontaminated soap applied
	2. Scrubs hands and wrists	a. All surfaces scrubbed (at least 3 inches above wrists) b. Minimum of 2 minutes spent scrubbing
	3. Completes procedure aseptically	a. Clean towel used for drying b. Water turned off without contaminating hands

SSE 1.2 Maintaining Asepsis		
Performance	**Essential Tasks**	**Evaluation Criteria**
A. Maintain Asepsis	1. Washes hands	a. Performed according to **SSE 1.1** b. Performed before and after procedure c. Performed whenever contamination is suspected
	2. Takes universal precautions	a. Performed whenever risk of exposure to body fluids exists b. Gloves, mask, and eye protection worn
	3. Uses aseptic technique	a. Only sterile or disinfected items obtained b. Items suspected of contamination replaced
	4. Performs procedure aseptically	a. Care used to avoid contaminating hands and items b. Repeats hand washing as needed

SSE 1.3
Isolation Technique

Performance	Essential Tasks	Evaluation Criteria
A. Prepare for Isolation	1. Maintains asepsis	a. Performed according to **SSE 1.2** b. Universal precautions followed
	2. Puts on isolation attire: • Hair covering • Mask • Eye coverings • Shoe coverings • Gown • Gloves	a. Performed correctly for procedure **(SOP)** b. Performed in sequence listed c. Performed without contaminating items d. Performed before entering room
	3. Administers prescribed therapy	a. Performed according to criteria for prescribed procedure
	4. Maintains equipment	a. Disposable items placed in proper receptacle b. Nondisposable items double bagged and labeled
	5. Removes isolation attire: • Shoe coverings • Gloves • Gown • Mask • Hair covering • Eye covering	a. Performed in sequence listed b. Performed without contaminating self c. Performed before leaving room (except in protective situations)

SSE 1.4
Equipment Cleaning

Performance	Essential Tasks	Evaluation Criteria
A. Clean Equipment	1. Takes universal precautions	a. Performed whenever risk of exposure to body fluids exists b. Gloves, mask, and eye protection worn
	2. Prepares equipment	a. Disposable items discarded b. Equipment disassembled c. Gloves worn
	3. Washes items	a. All debris removed
	4. Rinses items	a. All soap removed
	5. Dries items	a. Performed on all items to be sterilized b. All items dried thoroughly c. Potential heat damage avoided

Module 2.0

Basic Patient Assessment

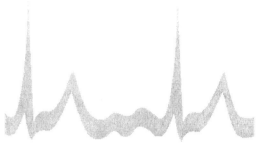

Respiratory care practitioners must be proficient in the skills required for routine data collection activities. Ordinarily, it is necessary to assess the patient's status before, during and following the administration of respiratory therapy. There are occasions when the patient's condition may preclude the initiation of prescribed therapy. On other occasions, changes in the patient's condition during therapy may necessitate discontinuing a procedure. The practitioner must also be aware of the patient's response to therapy, either positive or negative, in order to assist the physician in determining the course of treatment. This module addresses some of the basic data collection techniques which are routinely employed in conjunction with the delivery of respiratory care.

Objectives

Upon completion of this module, you will be able to:

1. Describe the rationale for routine implementation of basic patient assessment procedures.

2. Describe the patient characteristics which should be monitored through systematic observation techniques.

3. Collect and interpret vital sign data.

4. Collect and interpret respiratory data obtainable through chest auscultation.

Many of the characteristics of the patient's condition may be detected by a careful and skilled observer. These characteristics include the patient's physical appearance, respiratory status and apparent mental or emotional state. It is important to be able to detect abnormal characteristics that may exist at the time of initial contact with the patient along with changes which may occur during therapy. Although many observation skills can only be fully acquired through experience, it is first necessary to become thoroughly familiar with the relevant patient characteristics to be monitored.

Relevant physical attributes which may be of significance include edema, hives, rashes and abnormal skin tones. Edema results from general or localized retention of fluids and may indicate something as significant as congestive heart failure. The presence of hives or a rash may be a sign of an allergic reaction, often to a medication being administered. Cyanosis, or an ashen skin color, may be a sign of hypoxia. Flushing of the skin may indicate such conditions as fever, impaired circulation or hypertension. Whenever these conditions are observed, whether before or as a result of therapy, the nurse and/or physician and your supervisor should be notified.

Of particular concern to the respiratory therapy practitioner is the respiratory status of the patient. The primary indicator of respiratory status that is readily observable is breathing pattern. The pattern includes such variables as rate, depth and rhythm of breathing. The practitioner should always be on the alert for abnormal or rapidly changing breathing characteristics. Further discussion of this important topic will be delayed until the section on vital signs.

Changes in the patient's mental or emotional status should also be noted. If the patient exhibits any signs of confusion, slurred speech, visual disturbances, decreased attention span or impaired level of consciousness, the nurse and/or physician and your supervisor should be notified. These patient conditions may be attributed to factors such as reactions to drug therapy or changes in the patient's physical status and may require immediate attention.

The remainder of this module is devoted to patient assessment considerations related to vital signs and chest auscultation. Vital signs are taken routinely in conjunction with all types of respiratory therapy. Chest auscultation provides important information regarding the presence of secretions or obstructions in the airway. Because of the simplicity and frequency of performing these basic assessment procedures, the practitioner should be thoroughly familiar with the reasons for, and methods of, performing them.

Support Skill 2.1
Vital Signs

Heart rate, respiratory rate, blood pressure and body temperature have traditionally been considered patient vital signs. Respiratory therapy personnel routinely monitor heart and respiratory rates. Because blood pressure is monitored only occasionally and temperature determined rarely, if ever, as a part of the administration of respiratory therapy, the following discussion will be limited to the monitoring of pulse and respiration.

Heart or pulse rate is the number of ventricular contractions of the heart in one minute. A normal pulse rate is approximately 60 to 80 beats per minute. Heart rate is monitored either by auscultating the heart and counting the number of audible contractions or by placing the index and middle fingers over an artery and counting the number of palpations. For reliable results, the pulse rate should be monitored for at least one minute.

In order to assess patient response to therapy, pulse rate should always be monitored before, during and after the administration of therapy. Some patients receiving respiratory therapy may experience tachycardia. Factors contributing to this increased heart rate include hypoxemia, hypoxia, hyperventilation, reaction to medications and anxiety. Hyperventilation and anxiety may often be eliminated or greatly reduced by informing the patient about the procedure to be performed. Any time a pulse rate as great as 120 beats per minute is detected, or the rate increases by 20% or more, intermittent respiratory therapy procedures should be stopped and the physician notified.

Respiratory rate is the number of breaths taken in one minute. A normal respiratory rate is approximately 12 to 16 breaths per minute. Ordinarily, breathing is an involuntary function controlled by the autonomic nervous system. When individuals are aware of their breathing, however, they tend to increase their respiratory rate. Therefore, you should attempt to monitor the respiratory rate without the patient's awareness. This is best done by watching the rise and fall of the chest while holding the patient's wrist as if still monitoring the radial pulse. If the patient has extremely shallow respirations and you are unable to discern chest movement, it may be necessary for you to place your hand on the patient's chest in order to determine the respiratory rate.

Respiratory rate should also be monitored before, during and after all therapy. Since rapid respirations increase the work of breathing, patients should be encouraged to breathe slowly, maintaining an I:E ratio greater than 1:1. Anxiety and dyspnea are two of the primary factors contributing to increased respiratory rate. Again, properly informing the patient about the procedure to be performed can often eliminate or greatly reduce these factors.

Procedure for Monitoring Vital Signs

The following procedure is suggested for obtaining data related to patient vital signs:

1. Determine the heart rate by:

   a. Placing the index and middle fingers over the radial artery or placing the diaphragm of a stethoscope over the apex of the heart.

   b. Counting the number of ventricular contractions per minute.

2. Determine the respiratory rate by:

   a. Assuming a position where respirations can either be seen or felt.

   b. Unobtrusively counting the number of inhalations per minute.

3. During the administration of intermittent therapy, reassess the heart and respiratory rates at five-minute intervals.

Support Skill 2.2
Chest Auscultation

Faint sounds are produced during inspiration and expiration by the flow of air through the passages of the airway. These "normal" breath sounds result from the varying diameters and angulations of the passages through which the air must travel. The presence of obstructions or secretions in the airway will cause abnormal breath sounds to be produced. It is important for the respiratory therapy practitioner to be able to distinguish between normal and abnormal breath sounds.

The process of listening to breath sounds with the aid of a stethoscope is known as chest auscultation. The ability to distinguish normal from abnormal breath sounds takes much practice. Since mastery in interpreting sounds will greatly aid in identifying abnormal sounds, it is suggested that the beginner first practice auscultation on healthy individuals of normal or below normal body weight. Sounds normally heard over the chest wall are briefly described in *Table 2-1* on the following page.

It is quite difficult to describe adventitious or abnormal sounds adequately. For this reason, only the three most common adventitious sounds (rhonchi, rales and pleural friction rubs) will be discussed. For more information regarding chest auscultation terms, review the report from the Joint Committee of the American Thoracic Society referenced at the end of this section.

Rhonchi (wheezes) are high-pitched musical sounds heard predominantly on expiration. They are indicative of constriction of the airways or intralumi nal obstruction. They occur in all patients with obstructive lung disease, but are most predominant in asthmatics.

Rales are moist, "crackling" sounds heard mainly during inspiration. They are often compared with the sounds of crumpling cellophane or rubbing a few strands of hair between your fingers. Rales are indicative of airway secretions and may disappear or decrease in intensity following a cough.

A pleural rub is a creaky, leathery sound heard at end-inspiration and the beginning of expiration. This sound is created when inflamed pleural linings rub against each other. Frequently, the patient will complain of pain or discomfort over the inflamed area of the chest.

Whenever possible, the patient should be placed in an upright position to facilitate assessment of the entire chest wall. Since clothing tends to distort breath sounds, the best results will be obtained when chest auscul-

LOCATION AND DESCRIPTION
OF NORMAL BREATH SOUNDS

BREATH SOUND	LOCATION	DESCRIPTION
Tracheal	Over the trachea.	Identical, high-pitched, loud, inpiratory and expiratory sounds with a gap between end-inspiration and the beginning of expiration.
Bronchial	Over the main.	Identical, slightly stem bronchi lower-pitched, loud inspiratory and expiratory sounds with a gap between end-inspiration and the beginning of expiration.
Bronchovesicular	Over the major central airways and the right upper lobe apex.	Slightly muffled, medium pitched sounds heard on both inspiration and expiration.
Vesicular	Over the lung parenchyma, except the right upper lobe apex.	Moderately-pitched, "breezy" sounds heard on inspiration; fainter expiratory sounds.

Table 2-1.

tation is done over the bare chest. This means that clothing over the chest should be removed or loosened before performing chest auscultation.

It is sometimes easier to detect abnormal breath sounds by listening to and comparing symmetrical areas of the lung. Therefore, auscultation should be performed by listening over approximately the same area on both sides of the chest. Since asymmetrical breath sounds may also result from surgical procedures, such as lobectomy or chest tube insertion, the chest should be inspected for any scars or dressings signifying any of these surgical procedures.

Procedure for Chest Auscultation

When performing chest auscultation procedures, the following steps are recommended:

1.   Place the patient in an upright position.

2.   Inspect the chest for significant physical findings, such as scars, dressings and asymmetry.

3.   Instruct the patient to breathe slowly and deeply through the mouth.

4.   Place the diaphragm of the stethoscope on the patient's chest in the order indicated by the numbers in *Figure 2-1.*

5.   Listen to a full respiratory cycle before changing positions.

6.   Auscultate and compare symmetrical areas of the lungs by listening over the same area on both sides of the chest.

7.   Localize any adventitious breath sounds (rales, rhonchi or pleural friction rubs).

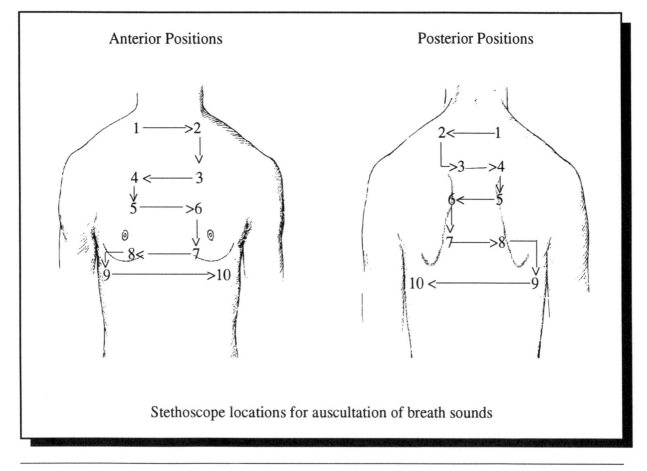

Stethoscope locations for auscultation of breath sounds

Evaluation of Basic Assessment Skills

The following definitions are provided for use whenever the respective Basic Assessment Support Skills are evaluated during the performance of a Clinical or Ancillary Procedure. In order for performance of the skills to be considered acceptable, all Essential Tasks are to be performed according to the accompanying Evaluation Criteria. Any deviation from the following task sequence or criteria must be approved by the evaluator.

SSE 2.1 Vital Signs		
Performance	**Essential Tasks**	**Evaluation Criteria**
A. Check Vital Signs	1. Determines heart rate	a. Index and middle finger or stethoscope correctly positioned. b. Counted for at least one (1) minute c. Rate computed accurately
	2. Determines respiratory rate	a. Performed unobtrusively (no apparent change in rate during assessment) b. Counted for at least one (1) minute
	3. Collects data as needed	a. Collected before performing procedure b. Collected after performing procedure c. Collected at minimum of 5-minute intervals during intermittent therapy

SSE 2.2 Chest Auscultation		
Performance	**Essential Tasks**	**Evaluation Criteria**
A. Auscultate Chest	1. Prepares patient	a. Placed in upright position (if possible) b. Clothing removed or loosened to enable auscultation on bare skin c. Proper breathing instructions provided (slowly and deeply)
	2. Inspects chest for: • Scars • Dressings • Asymmetry	a. Potential contributors to abnormal breath sounds identified
	3. Performs auscultation	a. Diaphragm of stethoscope correctly positioned b. Full respiratory cycle auscultated at each location c. All necessary locations auscultated d. Locations auscultated in correct sequence

Module 3.0

Data Management

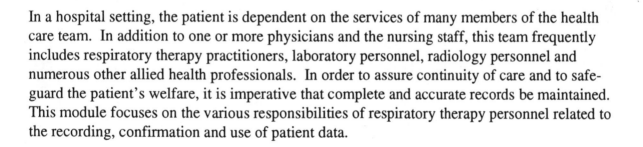

In a hospital setting, the patient is dependent on the services of many members of the health care team. In addition to one or more physicians and the nursing staff, this team frequently includes respiratory therapy practitioners, laboratory personnel, radiology personnel and numerous other allied health professionals. In order to assure continuity of care and to safeguard the patient's welfare, it is imperative that complete and accurate records be maintained. This module focuses on the various responsibilities of respiratory therapy personnel related to the recording, confirmation and use of patient data.

Objectives

Upon completion of this module, you will be able to:

1. Describe the importance of recording and using the data which appears on a patient's chart.

2. Review a patient's chart and select data which is pertinent to the prescribed therapy.

3. Ensure that the correct procedure is performed on the correct patient.

4. Record the results of respiratory therapy administration on a patient's chart.

Support Skill 3.1
Order Confirmation

A major risk associated with the administration of any therapy is that of human error. One potential source of error is the administration of different therapy, or administering the therapy in a different manner, than intended by the physician. Therefore, no therapy should be administered until the order is properly confirmed and the meaning of the order is fully understood.

A physician's order for respiratory therapy is usually communicated to the department by means of a requisition. This requisition must be confirmed by carefully comparing it with the original physician's order. Following confirmation, the order is then transcribed into a respiratory care plan. Since mistakes can be made in transcribing, the physician's order should be checked each time therapy is administered.

Occasionally, an order may be incomplete. For example, a physician may write an order for IPPB therapy indicating the tidal volume, FIO_2, medication and dosage, but omit the frequency of therapy. In such situations, it is necessary to initiate notification of the physician. Depending on hospital policy, you may be able to contact the physician yourself or it may be necessary to go through the nurse or your respiratory therapy supervisor.

There may be instances when all or a portion of the physician's order may be unfamiliar to you. When this occurs, the accuracy of the order must be questioned. The first step in this process is to discuss the order with your respiratory therapy supervisor. If your supervisor is also unfamiliar with the order, it will be necessary to obtain clarification from the physician.

Procedure for Confirming an Order

The following steps are suggested for confirming a respiratory care order:

1. Compare the requisition with the physician's order to ensure that no discrepancies exist.

2. Review the order to ensure that the following are prescribed:

   - Type of therapy
   - Frequency of therapy
   - Medication and dosage if required
   - Control parameters (e.g., FIO_2) if required for the prescribed therapy

3. If any part of the order is unfamiliar, question its accuracy.

Support Skill 3.2
Chart Review

An individual chart is maintained for each patient who is admitted to a hospital. The chart contains patient history and physical examination information, laboratory and radiology data, physician orders, progress notes and other diagnostic and therapeutic information. To aid in locating information, most patient charts are indexed with either tabs or colored paper. Before administering therapy to a patient, the respiratory therapy practitioner should review and extract all pertinent information.

The physician is responsible for completing the history and physical section of the chart. This section provides a brief record of the patient's family and personal health history and the results of the most recent physical examination, usually on the day of admittance. The physician is also responsible for including all orders for treatment and for maintaining continuous progress notes. The progress notes generally contain a description of all treatment plans accompanied by changes in patient status and other pertinent data related to the diagnosis and response to treatment.

Data obtained from the history and physical section and from the progress notes may suggest checking other portions of the chart for additional information. For instance, the patient may have an admitting diagnosis of pneumonia. To obtain information regarding the location of the pulmonary consolidation, it is necessary to consult the radiology section of the chart. Information related to the specific type of pneumonia present may be provided by the laboratory data. Review of the entire chart will enable you to determine the indications, contraindications and hazards for the prescribed therapy. This information will assist you in performing your duties in a responsible manner.

Procedure for Reviewing a Chart

When reviewing a patient's chart, it is recommended that the following tasks be performed:

1. On the patient's chart, identify all pertinent data in the following areas:

   • History and physical
   • Admitting diagnosis
   • Progress notes

2. Whenever indicated by the information obtained in performing the previous step, review the following sections of the chart:

   - Radiology reports
   - Laboratory reports
   - Blood gas analysis
   - Pulmonary function studies

3. Based on the data obtained, identify patient or other conditions that:

   - Indicate a need for the therapy
   - Contraindicate the therapy
   - Constitute potential hazards for the therapy

Support Skill 3.3
Patient Confirmation

It is essential to ensure that the prescribed therapy is administered to the correct patient. This process involves comparison of the room number and the patient name with the information found on the respiratory care order. If the hospital posts the patient's name on the door or bed, or both, it should match the name on the order. In addition, the patient should be checked personally by reading the name on the wristband and by greeting the patient by name. In addition to providing further confirmation, the greeting will aid in establishing and maintaining rapport with the patient. With all of these alternative procedures for identifying the patient, it is inexcusable for therapy to be administered to the wrong person.

Procedure for Confirming the Patient

It is recommended that the following steps be employed to ensure that the procedure is performed on the correct patient:

1. Match the information on the order with each of the following:

    • Room number
    • Name on the door or bed
    • Name on the wristband

2. Greet the patient by name (in a questioning manner if unknown).

3. Resolve any discrepancies in the patient identification information by conferring with the nursing staff.

Support Skill 3.4
Recording Results

The patient chart provides a legal record of the patient's response to therapy. Respiratory therapy personnel are responsible for ensuring that the results of all therapy are assessed and properly recorded. It is essential that all data be recorded accurately and completely.

Data recorded on the chart should relate only to therapy that has been recently administered. Charting should never be done before the administration of therapy has been completed. Furthermore, all charting should be done by the same individual who administered the therapy. All data is to be recorded in ink, the color determined by hospital policy. If an error is made while charting, a single line should be drawn through the error and the error initialed. Finally, the chart should be signed using the initial of the first name and the full last name.

Occasionally, a pertinent patient observation that is unrelated to the therapy may be made. Such information should be communicated directly to the nurse and/or physician, as appropriate, and to your supervisor.

Procedure for Recording Results

When recording results, the following procedure is recommended:

1. Record the following data on the patient's chart:

   - Date
   - Time
   - Pulse rate
   - Respiratory rate
   - Abnormal physical characteristics
   - Therapy-related patient complaints
   - Amount, color and consistency of sputum produced

2. Sign the patient chart (first initial and full last name).

Evaluation of Data Management Skills

The following definitions are provided for use whenever the respective Data Management Support Skills are evaluated during the performance of a Clinical or Ancillary Procedure. In order for performance of the skills to be considered acceptable, all Essential Tasks are to be performed according to the accompanying Evaluation Criteria. Any deviation from the following task sequence or criteria must be approved by the evaluator.

SSE 3.1 Order Confirmation		
Performance	**Essential Tasks**	**Evaluation Criteria**
A. Check Order	1. Compares requisition with order	a. All discrepancies identified b. All discrepancies rectified before continuing
	2. Ensures completeness of order	a. All missing information noted b. All missing information obtained before continuing
	3. Questions unfamiliar content of order	a. Procedure delayed until questions are resolved

SSE 3.2 Chart Review		
Performance	**Essential Tasks**	**Evaluation Criteria**
A. Review Chart	1. Identifies pertinent data in the: • History and physical • Admitting diagnosis • Progress notes	a. All pertinent data identified for the evaluator
	2. Reviews relevant data in the: • Radiology reports • Laboratory reports • Blood gas analysis • Pulmonary function studies	a. All relevant data identified and reviewed with the evaluator
	3. Draws conclusions regarding: • Indications • Contraindications • Hazards	a. Indications described accurately b. Hazards and contraindications described accurately c. Appropriate actions to minimize hazards explained

SSE 3.3 Patient Confirmation		
Performance	**Essentials Tasks**	**Evaluation Criteria**
A. Confirm Patient	1. Identifies patient by: • Checking room number • Checking name on door and/or bed • Checking wristband • Greeting patient by name	a. All steps performed b. Any discrepancies identified
	2. Resolves discrepancies	a. Nursing staff contacted b. Procedure delayed until correct patient confirmed

SSE 3.4
Recording Results

Performance	Essential Tasks	Evaluation Criteria
A. Record Results	1. Records the following patients data: • Date • Time • Type of therapy • Pulse rate • Respiratory rate • Abnormal physical characteristics • Therapy-related complaints • Sputum characteristics	a. Only factual information charted b. No important details omitted c. No irrelevant data recorded d. All information accurate e. All errors properly corrected
	2. Sign patient chart	a. First inital and full last name used

Module 4.0

Communication Skills

The quality of respiratory care is often influenced by the ability of practitioners to communicate both with patients and with other clinical personnel. The necessary communication skills include more than just the ability to verbally transmit and receive information. The manner of communicating with others may have an equally important effect upon the quality of care provided. This module addresses the interpersonal communication skills which appear to relate most directly to the administration of respiratory therapy.

Objectives

Upon completion of this module, you will be able to:

1. Describe the importance of effective communication skills for respiratory therapy personnel.

2. Explain to a patient the purpose and method of performing a respiratory therapy procedure and what is expected of the patient during the procedure.

3. Improve patient rapport and cooperation through the effective use of communication skills.

4. Effectively communicate with other hospital personnel regarding patient welfare.

The effectiveness of communication depends upon the clarity of the transmitted message, the ability of the receiver of the message to listen effectively and the interpersonal relationship between the two parties involved. An inadequacy in any one or more of these areas will prevent successful communication from taking place.

The clarity of the message is influenced by several factors. First, the vocabulary used must be appropriate for the listener. A precise technical vocabulary may be essential for communicating with other health professionals, but use of the same terminology with patients may inhibit understanding. In addition, technical jargon may cause a patient to "turn off" to the conversation.

A related factor is the organization of the message being transmitted. If information is presented in a lengthy, rambling manner with important ideas omitted or jumbled, the listener will only be confused. A final factor is the clarity of the speaker's voice. Words are wasted if they are poorly articulated, spoken so fast that they run together or spoken too softly.

For effective communication, good listening skills are just as important as good speaking skills. This applies both to health professionals and to patients. To obtain accurate information regarding a patient's condition, it is often necessary to listen both attentively and analytically. It may also be necessary to ask clarifying questions in order to ensure understanding. Special efforts may also be necessary to ensure patient understanding of your message. This is particularly true for patients who are partially sedated or confused because of their physical or mental state.

The third area identified as influencing the effectiveness of communication is the interpersonal relationship between the speaker and the listener. This idea encompasses a number of related factors. Of particular importance is the attitude of the speaker. A lack of concern or a feeling of superiority or inferiority is surely to be communicated, either nonverbally or by the tone and manner of verbal expression. For successful communication with patients, the development of trust and rapport is imperative.

In this module, there will be no attempt to provide a comprehensive treatment of communication skills and their application. Instead, we will focus our attention on certain types of interaction which are essential components of many respiratory therapy procedures. Our discussion of communication skills will be organized according to their use when interacting with patients and when interacting with other personnel.

Two types of patient interaction situations frequently occur during the administration of therapy. These situations are: (1) informing the patient of the procedure to be performed and (2) reassuring the patient during and following the therapy. Only one personnel interaction situation has been built into the evaluation procedures. That situation is the reporting of patient or therapy-related information to appropriate health professionals.

Support Skill 4.1
Informing the Patient

This Support Skill has been included as an essential element of most respiratory therapy procedures because of its importance to the success of the therapy. The primary purpose of this activity is to secure the cooperation of the patient. Because of the positive influence that patient cooperation exerts on most types of respiratory therapy, all practitioners should develop proficiency in the skill of informing the patient.

One aspect of informing the patient should be obvious. It is the process of communicating the purpose, method and frequency of performing the therapeutic procedure. This information enables the patient to understand what to do and what to expect. Furthermore, the informed patient may be less fearful of the process and the consequences of the therapy. By alleviating fear and misunderstanding, the likelihood of patient cooperation is greatly enhanced.

The process of informing the patient also provides an opportunity for the practitioner to begin developing patient rapport. The manner in which the patient is informed, both verbally and nonverbally, will influence the trust and respect that the patient develops for the practitioner and will set the stage for further patient-practitioner interaction. The rapport that is established is a major factor in determining the level of patient cooperation during the administration of therapy.

Procedure for Informing the Patient

The following guidelines should be considered when informing the patient:

1. Introduce yourself by name and department (if not already acquainted).

2. Tell the patient what procedure is to be performed.

3. Explain the procedure by describing:

   - Why it is to be performed
   - How it will be performed
   - What the patient is expected to do
   - What you will be doing
   - How frequently it will be performed

4. Ask the patient if there are any questions regarding the procedure.

5. Answer any questions:

    • Accurately
    • At a level appropriate for the patient's ability to comprehend

Support Skill 4.2
Reassuring the Patient

When the patient is conscious, there will be some form of patient-practitioner interaction taking place throughout the administration of therapy. It is important that this interaction be used to build and maintain patient rapport. Just as patient cooperation is needed during an entire therapeutic procedure, efforts to gain this cooperation through effective communication must be a continuous process. The communication skills used to inform the patient should be applied during all patient interaction situations.

This Support Skill is referred to as "Reassuring the Patient" because that is exactly what many patients need. The hospital surroundings, unfamiliar equipment and nature of many respiratory therapy procedures may all create a frightening, even traumatic, experience for the patient. Therefore, the patient may need constant reassurance that the best of care is being provided. It is important that the patient believes that you and the other health professionals are competent and caring individuals. This impression is difficult to establish unless these qualities actually exist. If they exist, they can be communicated through sincerity and the conscientious performance of tasks.

Although each patient situation may be unique, there are some general guidelines which should help you identify specific actions that may be used in efforts to reassure the patient. Conversation which does not detract from the therapy is usually beneficial. The conversation should be appropriate to the age and other characteristics of the patient. It should be positive and include topics of interest to the patient. Frequent questions should be asked regarding patient needs and concern about the therapy. In addition, patients should be encouraged to ask questions related to their concerns. Questions should always be answered as honestly and as effectively as possible without violating any confidentiality. To build respect and credibility, every reasonable effort should be made to follow through on needs expressed by the patient.

As a final note, it should never be assumed that a patient cannot hear or understand. Even when administering therapy to a patient known to be comatose, your words and behavior should be the same as if the patient were alert. You can never be certain that the patient is totally unaware of what is being said nor when the patient may suddenly awaken or regain consciousness.

Procedure for Reassuring the Patient

The following procedure is recommended for reassuring the patient:

1. Whenever appropriate, attempt to conduct a positive, interesting conversation with the patient.

2. Explain the consequences of your actions in administering therapy, emphasizing:

    • The potential benefits
    • The importance of cooperation
    • Your intentions to be careful and to minimize pain or discomfort

3. Ask if the patient has any needs or questions (particularly at the conclusion of therapy).

4. Make every reasonable effort to satisfy the patient's needs.

5. Answer questions as effectively as possible.

Support Skill 4.3
Reporting Observations

Up to this point, the emphasis has been on communication and interaction with patients. There are also many circumstances involving interaction with peers, supervisors, physicians, nurses, other health professionals and various hospital support personnel. Although communication with these individuals will be different than with patients, the effectiveness of communication is equally important. The nature of this communication will not only affect the quality of care received by patients, but will also influence your satisfaction and security as an employee.

We will attempt to address all of the factors which influence your interaction with various hospital personnel. This Support Skill focuses upon the aspects of personnel communication which are most likely to affect the quality of patient care and which are often observable during the performance of a respiratory therapy procedure. Most of this communication is routine and occurs following completion of treatment.

As a follow-up to your interaction with the patient, important requests or complaints voiced by the patient should be transmitted to the nurse, physician or other appropriate personnel. In addition, any reactions to therapy or other pertinent observations of the patient, even though they may be recorded on the chart, should be communicated to the nurse and/or physician and your supervisor. Adverse reactions to therapy or other significant changes in the patient's condition should be reported immediately upon observation.

Procedure for Reporting Observations

The following procedure is recommended for reporting observations:

1. Report any significant adverse changes in the patient's condition to the nurse and/or physician and your supervisor whenever observed.

2. Following the procedure, inform the appropriate personnel of:

    • Patient requests
    • Patient complaints
    • Unexpressed patient needs

3.   Following the procedure, report to the nurse and/or physician and your supervisor:

   • Any non-critical adverse reactions to the therapy
   • Other pertinent observations of the patient's condition

Evaluation of Communication Skills

The following definitions are provided for use whenever the respective Communication Skills are evaluated during the performance of a Clinical or Ancillary Procedure. In order for performance of the skills to be considered acceptable, all Essential Tasks are to be performed according to the accompanying Evaluation Criteria. Any deviation from the following task sequence or criteria must be approved by the evaluator.

SSE 4.1 Informing the Patient		
Performance	**Essential Tasks**	**Evaluation Criteria**
A. Inform Patient	1. Provides information regarding: • Name and department • What procedure • Why performed • How performed • Patient responsibilities • How often performed	a. Complete information provided b. Accurate information provided c. Words spoken clearly d. Words spoken slowly e. No technical jargon used
	2. Assures patient understanding by: • Asking for questions • Answering questions effectively	a. Questions solicited as frequently as needed b. Information reworded when repeated c. Vocabulary adjusted as necessary d. Process continued until patient understands

SSE 4.2 Reassuring the Patient		
Proformance	**Essential Tasks**	**Evaluation Criteria**
A. Reassure Patient	1. Talks to patient to: • Establish rapport • Explain benefits of therapy • Explain need for cooperation • Obtain patient confidence • Reduce anxiety and fear	a. Efforts to involve patient in conversation attempted b. Friendly, cheerful approach used (e.g., smiled appropriately, used positive words, etc.) c. Efforts made to convey information d. Remained calm throughout
	2. Tends to patient needs	a. Patient asked regarding needs b. Obvious effort made to satisfy needs c. Questions answered accurately and completely

SSE 4.3 Reporting Observations		
Proformance	**Essential Tasks**	**Evaluation Criteria**
A. Report Observations	1. Reports significant adverse changes	a. Any adverse changes identified b. Changes reported immediately c. Changes reported to appropriate personnel
	2. Informs personnel of: • Patient requests • Patient complaints • Unexpressed patient needs • Non-critical reactions to therapy • Other pertinent observations	a. Unexpressed needs and conditions identified b. Reported following therapy c. Reported to appropriate personnel d. Reported according to protocol e. Reported accurately

Section Two
Ancillary Procedures

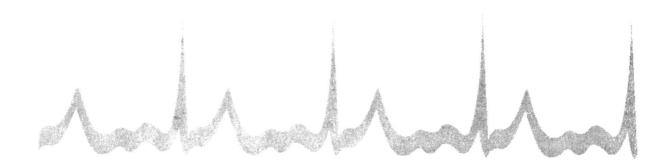

Module 5.0

Disinfection and Sterilization

In a hospital setting, considerable care must be taken to prevent the spread of infection by the use of contaminated equipment. In respiratory therapy, this type of cross-contamination is of particular concern because of the manner in which equipment is used. During use, most respiratory therapy equipment comes in direct contact with secretions and gases of the patient's respiratory system and is operated under conditions that provide a warm, moist environment that encourages bacterial growth. In addition, most of the equipment is transported throughout the hospital and reused by other patients. Unless this equipment is free from contamination before reuse, infection is likely to spread from patient to patient.

Objectives

Upon completion of this module, you will be able to complete the following:

1. Describe the importance of disinfection and sterilization procedures.

2. List the advantages and disadvantages of the various types of decontamination procedures.

3. Disinfect or sterilize respiratory therapy equipment by means of:

    • Chemical disinfection
    • Pasteurization
    • Steam autoclave sterilization
    • Ethylene oxide sterilization

The first step in the decontamination of respiratory therapy equipment is thorough washing or cleaning to remove any substances such as blood, secretions or other debris adhering to the surface. Universal precautions must be observed. The procedures for cleaning equipment are essentially the same, regardless of the procedure used for disinfection or sterilization. For this reason, the process of cleaning equipment is considered a Support Skill.

A variety of procedures are used to destroy or inhibit the growth of micro-organisms. Most of these procedures employ either high temperature or chemical action. Sterilization techniques kill microorganisms both in the active, growing stage and in the resting or spore stage. Disinfection procedures are only effective for destroying active, growing bacteria.

Because certain materials used in the manufacture of equipment may be damaged by either heat or chemicals, it is necessary to select sterilization procedures that can be tolerated best by the particular equipment to be sterilized. Whenever equipment tolerance is not a factor, selection of a sterilization procedure is usually governed by hospital policy. Factors influencing the selection of procedures include: characteristics of the equipment to be sterilized, cost of the sterilization equipment and supplies to be used and the time required to complete the process.

Ancillary Procedure 5.1
Chemical Disinfection

One of the simplest methods of killing bacteria is by immersing equipment in a chemical disinfectant. The most commonly used chemical for disinfecting equipment is the acid glutaraldehyde (i.e., Cidex). Unless equipment remains submerged in this chemical for an extended period of time, bacterial spores will not be killed. Therefore, this method is only used in hospital situations where disinfection of equipment is considered adequate.

Following disinfection, equipment should be thoroughly rinsed, dried and packaged under aseptic conditions. The fact that equipment is not packaged until after it is disinfected represents a major disadvantage of this procedure. Unless proper care is exercised prior to and during packaging, the equipment can easily become contaminated.

Chemical disinfection has been simplified by the development of an automatic decontamination system known as the Cidematic. Because this system automatically cleans and disinfects, it is not necessary to handle the equipment until it is ready to be dried, thus reducing the risk of contamination.

Procedure for Chemical Disinfection

The following procedure is recommended for the chemical disinfection of equipment:

A. *Clean Equipment.* Following universal precautions, disassemble, wash and rinse all equipment to be disinfected chemically.

B. *Immerse Equipment.* Completely submerge the equipment in the solution used for chemical disinfection, avoiding all air pockets. Allow the equipment to soak for the specified time (10 to 20 minutes).

C. *Rinse Items.* Aseptically remove the equipment from the solution and rinse it thoroughly to remove all traces of the chemical residue.

D. *Dry Items.* Aseptically dry the equipment by placing it under heat lamps or inside a drying cabinet.

E. *Assemble Equipment.* Aseptically reassemble the dry equipment according to the standard procedure of the hospital.

F. **Package Equipment.** Aseptically package the equipment according to the standard procedure of the hospital.

G. **Store Equipment.** Store the equipment in the designated storage area, maintaining rotation of stock.

Ancillary Procedure 5.2
Pasteurization

Another common method of disinfecting equipment is by pasteurization. In this method, equipment is immersed in hot water (170°F or 77°C) for 30 minutes. This procedure is relatively fast, inexpensive and safe for most pieces of equipment. The primary disadvantages of pasteurization are that spores are not killed by the process and equipment must be dried and packaged after disinfection, thereby risking possible contamination.

Procedure for Pasteurization

The following procedure is recommended for pasteurization:

A. *Clean Equipment*. Following universal precautions, disassemble, wash and rinse all equipment to be disinfected by pasteurization.

B. *Immerse Equipment*. Completely submerge the equipment in the hot water bath, avoiding all air pockets. Allow the equipment to soak for the specified time (30 minutes at 170°F).

C. *Dry Items*. Aseptically dry the equipment by placing it under heat lamps or inside a drying cabinet.

D. *Assemble Equipment*. Aseptically reassemble the dry equipment according to the standard procedure of the hospital.

E. *Package Equipment*. Aseptically package the equipment according to the standard procedure of the hospital.

F. *Store Equipment*. Store the equipment in the designated storage area, maintaining rotation of stock.

Ancillary Procedure 5.3
Steam Autoclave Sterilization

The most frequently used method of equipment sterilization is by means of the steam autoclave. This method is highly effective and efficient and is relatively inexpensive. This method utilizes pressurized steam to produce sufficiently high temperatures (250 to 270°F) to kill both active and dormant microorganisms. Because equipment is packaged and sealed before sterilization, it is not subject to contamination until opened for use. The major disadvantage of steam autoclave sterilization is that it cannot be used for equipment that is subject to the effects of high temperature.

Procedure for Steam Autoclave Sterilization

The following procedure is recommended for steam autoclave sterilization:

A. *Clean Equipment.* Following universal precautions, disassemble, wash, rinse and dry all equipment to be placed in the autoclave.

B. *Assemble Equipment.* Aseptically reassemble the dry equipment according to the standard procedure of the hospital.

C. *Package Equipment.* Package the equipment with linen or paper wrap according to the standard procedure of the hospital. Seal with steam autoclave sterilization tape.

D. *Label Packages.* Label the packages in terms of their contents, date sterilized, expiration date and batch number.

E. *Position Packages.* Position the packages in the autoclave to assure full exposure of the equipment and evaporation of moisture.

F. *Operate Autoclave.* Operate the autoclave according to the manufacturer's specifications.

G. *Store Equipment.* When the sterilization process is complete, remove the equipment from the sterilizer and store it in the designated storage area, maintaining rotation of stock.

Ancillary Procedure 5.4
Ethylene Oxide Sterlization

When performed properly, sterilization using ethylene oxide gas is highly effective in destroying both active and dormant microorganisms. Since ethylene oxide gas is highly toxic and flammable, caution must be exercised when performing this procedure. In order to protect the patient against the toxic effects of residues of ethylene oxide remaining on materials sterilized by this procedure, it is necessary to aerate equipment before patient use. Although certain plastic materials may be damaged by ethylene oxide, the procedure is relatively safe for most equipment and is useful for the sterilization of most equipment that is subject to the effects of high temperature.

Procedure for Ethylene Oxide Sterilization

The following procedure is recommended for ethylene oxide gas sterilization:

A.   *Clean Equipment*. Following universal precautions, disassemble, wash, rinse and dry all equipment to be sterilized with ethylene oxide.

B.   *Assemble Equipment*. Aseptically reassemble the dry equipment according to the standard procedure of the hospital.

C.   *Package Equipment*. Package the equipment with plastic or paper wrap according to the standard procedure of the hospital. Seal the package with ethylene oxide sterilization tape.

D.   *Label Packages*. Label the packages in terms of their contents, date sterilized, expiration date and batch number.

E.   *Position Packages*. Position the packages in the sterilizer in a manner that assures full exposure to the gas.

F.   *Operate Sterilizer*. Exercising caution in handling the ethylene oxide canister, operate the sterilizer according to the manufacturer's instructions.

G.   *Aerate Equipment*. When the sterilization cycle is complete, remove the equipment from the sterilizer and aerate it for the period of time that is appropriate for the equipment type and

Notes

aeration procedure. (Aeration chambers greatly reduce aeration time.)

H. **_Store Equipment_**. When the aeration cycle is complete, store the equipment in the designated storage area, maintaining rotation of stock.

Evaluation of Decontamination Procedures

The following definitions are provided for use whenever the respective Disinfection and Sterilization Procedures are evaluated. In order for performance of the procedures to be considered acceptable, all Essential Tasks are be performed according to the accompanying Evaluation Criteria. Any deviation from the following task sequence or criteria must be approved by the evaluator.

APE 5.1 Chemical Decontamination		
Performance	**Essential Tasks**	**Evaluation Criteria**
A. Clean Equipment	See SSE 1.4	See SSE 1.4
B. Immerse Equipment	1. Submerges equipment in solution	a. No parts exposed b. No air pockets c. Adequate soaking time (10-20 minutes)
C. Rinse Items	1. Removes equipment from solution 2. Rinses equipment with water	a. Aseptically (**SSE 1.2**) a. Aseptically (**SSE 1.2**) b. All chemical residue removed
D. Dry Items	1. Dries equipment by: Heat lamps, or Drying cabinets	a. Aseptically (**SSE 1.2**) b. Equipment thoroughly dried
E. Assemble Equipment	1. Reassemble all pieces or equipment	a. Aseptically (**SSE 1.2**) b. According to **SOP**
F. Package Equipment	1. Packages assembled equipment	a. Aseptically (**SSE 1.2**) b. According to **SOP**
G. Store Equipment	1. Places equipment in storage area	a. Placed in designated area b. Stock rotated

APE 5.2
Pasteurization

Performance	Essential Tasks	Evaluation Criteria
A. Clean Equipment	See SSE 1.4	See SSE 1.4
B. Immerse Equipment	1. Submerges equipment in hot water	a. 170°F b. No parts exposed c. Adequate soaking time (30 minutes)
C. Dry Items	1. Dries equipment by: Heat lamps, or Drying cabinets	a. Aseptically (SSE 1.2) b. Equipment thoroughly dried
D. Assemble Equipment	1. Reassembles all pieces of equipment	a. Aseptically (SSE 1.2) b. According to SOP
E. Package Equipment	1. Packages assembled equipment	a. Aseptically (SSE 1.2) b. According to SOP
F. Store Equipment	1. Places equipment in storage area	a. Placed in designated area b. Stock rotated

APE 5.3 Steam Autoclave Sterilization		
Performance	**Essential Tasks**	**Evaluation Criteria**
A. Clean Equipment	See **SSE 1.4**	See **SSE 1.4**
B. Assemble Equipment	1. Reassembles all pieces of equipment	a. Aseptically (**SSE 1.2**) b. According to **SOP**
C. Package Equipment	1. Wraps the equipment	a. Aseptically (**SSE 1.2**) b. According to **SOP** c. Linen or paper wrap used
	2. Seals the package	a. Steam autoclave tape used
D. Label Packages	1. Indicates sterilization information	a. Contents b. Date sterilized c. Expiration date d. Batch number
E. Position Packages	1. Places packages in autoclave	a. Full exposure to steam assured b. No-heat sensitive items inserted
F. Operate Autoclave	1. Operates steam autoclave	a. According to **SOP**
G. Store Equipment	1. Places equipment in storage area	a. Placed in designated area b. Stock rotated

APE 5.4 Ethylene Oxide Sterilization		
Performance	**Essential Tasks**	**Evaluation Criteria**
A. Clean Equipment	See SSE 1.4	See SSE 1.4
B. Assemble Equipment	1. Reassembles all pieces of equipment	a. Aseptically (**SSE 1.2**) b. According to **SOP**
C. Package Equipment	1. Wraps the equipment	a. Aseptically (**SSE 1.2**) b. According to **SOP** c. Plastic or paper wrap used
	2. Seals the package	a. Ethylene oxide tape used
D. Label Packages	1. Indicates sterilization information.	a. Contents b. Date sterilized c. Expiration date d. Batch number
E. Position Packages	1. Places packages in gas autoclave	a. Full exposure to gas assured b. No ethylene oxide sensitive items inserted
F. Operate Sterilizer	1. Operates ethylene oxide sterilizer	a. According to **SOP** b. Handles ethylene oxide canister with caution
G. Aerate Equipment	1. Removes equipment from sterilizer	a. Aseptically (**SSE 1.2**)
	2. Aerates equipment according to type	a. According to **SOP** b. Ethylene oxide removed
H. Store Equipment	1. Places equipment in storage area	a. Placed in designated area b. Stock rotated

Module 6.0

Advanced Patient Assessment

An earlier module presented several basic assessment procedures that are routinely performed with patients receiving respiratory care. The present module addresses procedures of a more complex and specialized nature that are frequently required in order to determine respiratory status. These procedures include ventilatory assessment, arterial blood sampling, and noninvasive blood gas monitoring.

Ventilatory assessment includes the measurement of tidal volume, minute ventilation, forced vital capacity, and maximum inspiratory pressure. Arterial blood sampling pertains to the collection of a sample for blood gas analysis. Noninvasive blood gas monitoring refers to the procedures of pulse oximetry, capnography, and transcutaneous monitoring.

Objectives

Upon completion of this module, you will be able to:

1. Explain the rationale for assessment of ventilatory status.

2. Using a simple spirometer, measure tidal volume, minute ventilation, and forced vital capacity.

3. Using a pressure manometer, measure maximum inspiratory pressure.

4. Describe the indications for the collection of an arterial blood sample.

5. Perform the procedures required for arterial blood sampling.

6. Discuss the rationale behind noninvasive blood gas monitoring.

7. Using a pulse oximeter, measure oxygen saturation.

8. Using a capnograph, measure exhaled carbon dioxide levels.

9. Using a transcutaneous monitor, measure oxygen and carbon dioxide levels.

Ancillary Procedure 6.1
Ventilatory Assessment

Proper respiratory care often requires information regarding a patient's ability to breathe spontaneously without ventilatory assistance. The maintenance of adequate respiration requires that an individual be able to increase the rate and depth of breathing as necessary without experiencing fatigue or an increase in the *work of breathing*. Unless the patient has an adequate ventilatory reserve, a life-threatening condition of respiratory distress can result.

The presence of respiratory distress can be detected by assessing ventilatory mechanics. Such distress may or may not be accompanied by dyspnea. Some patients may appear very distressed, yet have normal or near normal ventilatory parameters. Other patients, especially those with COPD, may experience no labored breathing, yet have inadequate pulmonary function. Therefore, it is imperative that procedures for determining the patient's true ventilatory status be performed.

The ventilatory mechanics of potential victims of respiratory distress are assessed frequently to detect changes in status and to determine if continuous mechanical ventilation is indicated. Patients already receiving mechanical ventilation are monitored routinely to determine when they are able to breathe without assistance. This assessment must be continued while weaning a patient from continuous mechanical ventilation in order to follow the patient's progress in becoming independent of mechanical ventilation.

Ventilatory Parameters

The patient's ventilatory reserve can be estimated from data obtained by simple bedside assessment procedures. This assessment includes the determination of tidal volume, minute ventilation, and forced vital capacity by means of bedside spirometry and the measurement of maximum inspiratory pressure using a pressure manometer.

Tidal Volume (V_T)

The tidal volume of a patient can be obtained by having the patient maintain a regular respiratory pattern while breathing through a simple spirometer. For the sake of reliability, it is recommended that the tidal volume be determined by averaging the expired volume over the period of a minute. Tidal volume can be determined as a calculation of minute ventilation. In order to maintain adequate ventilation without assistance, the tidal volume should ordinarily be at least 4 to 5 ml/kg of the patient's body weight.

Minute Ventilation ($\dot{V}_E$)

A simple spirometer can be used to measure minute ventilation. Minute ventilation is measured by having the patient breathe normally while exhaling through the spirometer for one minute. During that time period, the respiratory rate is counted. The total amount of exhaled gas in a minute equals the minute ventilation. By dividing minute ventilation by the respiratory rate, average tidal volume is calculated. Normal minute ventilation is considered to be 5 to 10 l/m.

Forced Vital Capacity (FVC)

A simple spirometer can also be used to measure vital capacity. To provide an indication of a patient's ventilatory reserve under stress, a measure of vital capacity under forced conditions is usually obtained. The forced vital capacity is measured by having the patient inspire maximally and exhale through the spirometer as quickly and completely as possible. Ventilatory assistance may be indicated whenever the vital capacity is less than 10 to 15 ml/kg body weight.

Maximal Inspiratory Pressure (MIP)

To maintain an adequate vital capacity, the patient must possess the minimum acceptable level of respiratory muscle strength. This strength is reflected by a measure of maximal inspiratory pressure (also referred to as negative inspiratory force and peak inspiratory pressure) as measured by a pressure manometer. The patient should have sufficient muscle strength to exert a maximal inspiratory pressure of at least -20 cm H_2O. When forced vital capacity cannot be measured, MIP can be used to estimate the patient's ventilatory reserve.

Procedure for Assessing Ventilatory Status

It is suggested that a bedside ventilatory assessment procedure be performed in the following manner:

A. *Maintain Asepsis.* While performing the remainder of this procedure, you are expected to maintain aseptic conditions and follow universal precautions according to the procedure described in **SSE 1.2**. This includes washing your hands:

   • Before obtaining equipment
   • Following performance of *I. Conclude Procedure*
   • Anytime during the procedure that contamination is suspected

B. *Prepare Equipment.* Obtain and assemble the following equipment:

   • Portable spirometer and patient attachment
   • Negative pressure manometer and patient attachment

C. *Confirm Patient.* Ensure that the procedure is performed with the correct patient as follows:

   1. Match the information on the order with the following:

      • Room number
      • Name on the door or bed
      • Name on the wristband

   2. Greet the patient by name (in a questioning manner if unknown).

   3. Resolve any discrepancies in the patient identification information by conferring with the nursing staff.

D. *Inform Patient.* Interact with the patient as follows:

   1. Introduce yourself by name and department (if not already acquainted).

   2. Tell the patient what procedure is to be performed.

   3. Explain the procedure by describing:

      • Why it is to be performed
      • How it will be performed
      • What the patient is expected to do
      • What you will be doing
      • How frequently it will be performed

E. *Demonstrate FVC, V_T and $\dot{V}_E$ Procedures.* Describe and demonstrate the following:

1. Procedure for using the spirometer (simulate demonstration).

2. Normal tidal volume breathing.

3. Maximal inspiration followed by rapid and complete exhalation.

F. *Implement FVC, V_T and $\dot{V}_E$ Procedures.* Perform the following tasks:

1. Position the patient in an upright position (45 to 90°).

2. Connect the patient to the spirometer with the appropriate attachment (if a mouthpiece is used, attach noseclips).

3. Instruct the patient to breathe normally through the spirometer for sixty seconds.

4. Determine respiratory rate and minute ventilation and calculate the patient's tidal volume by dividing the $\dot{V}_E$ by the total rate.

5. Encourage the patient to perform the FVC procedure as demonstrated.

6. Read and record the patient's forced vital capacity.

7. Repeat the FVC procedure at least three times, allowing the patient sufficient rest between performances.

8. Select and record the FVC value for the patient's best effort.

G. *Demonstrate MIP Procedure.* Describe and demonstrate the following:

1. Procedure for using the manometer set-up (simulate demonstration).

2. Maximal exhalation followed by maximal inhalation.

H. *Implement MIP Procedure.* Perform the following tasks:

1. Connect the patient to the pressure manometer with the appropriate attachment (if a mouthpiece is used, attach noseclips).

2. Encourage the patient to perform the MIP procedure as demonstrated.

3. Read and record the patient's maximal inspiratory pressure.

4. Repeat the MIP procedure at least three times, allowing the patient sufficient rest between performances.

5. Select and record the MIP value for the patient's best effort.

I. *Conclude Procedure.* Complete the following tasks:

1. Place the patient in a comfortable position.

2. Assure that the call bell and bedside table are within the patient's reach.

3. Unplug and cover the equipment and move it away from the patient's bedside (or remove it from the room).

4. Ask if the patient has any needs.

5. Answer any questions as effectively as possible.

J. **Record Results.** Document the therapy as follows:

1. Record the following data on the patient's chart:

    *   Date
    *   Time
    *   Tidal volume
    *   Minute ventilation
    *   Forced vital capacity
    *   MIP
    *   Abnormal patient characteristics
    *   Therapy-related patient complaints

2. Sign the patient's chart (first initial and full last name).

K. *Report Observations.* Report the following information:

1. Report any significant adverse changes in the patient's condition to the nurse or physician whenever observed.

2. Following the procedure, inform the appropriate personnel of:

    *   Patient requests
    *   Patient complaints
    *   Unexpressed patient needs

3. Following the procedure, report to the nurse or physician:

    *   Any non-critical adverse reactions to the therapy
    *   Other pertinent observations of the patient's condition

Ancillary Procedure 6.2
Arterial Blood Sampling

The acid-base balance and ventilatory status of a patient can be determined by analyzing a sample of arterial blood. Both metabolic and respiratory disorders can be identified in this way. Such an analysis is essential for determining the origin of a disorder so that proper treatment can be provided. The procedure for collecting an arterial blood sample for analysis is the topic of the present discussion. Universal precautions must always be followed when collecting blood samples and when handling the sample and the syringe.

Arterial blood is sampled by inserting the needle of a syringe directly into an artery. Prepackaged blood gas kits are most commonly used for collecting a sample of arterial blood. Such kits contain a heparinized syringe, an assortment of needle sizes, a needle cap, skin preparation pads, a gauze pad, and an ice container.

If a blood gas kit is not available, it is recommended that a glass syringe be used for collecting the sample. In addition to being impermeable to gas, a glass syringe has a plunger which moves freely inside the barrel. Because of the free movement, the pressure of arterial blood is usually sufficient to fill the syringe. If a plastic syringe is used, it is usually necessary to aspirate the blood by withdrawing the plunger manually in order to fill the syringe. This action introduces the risk of obtaining venous blood by mistake.

To prevent the blood sample from clotting before and during analysis, a blood gas kit contains a heparinized syringe. If it is necessary to use an ordinary glass syringe, it is important to coat the inside of the syringe and needle with an anticoagulant. In addition to preventing the sample from clotting, the anticoagulant lubricates the plunger allowing it to slide more freely. The anticoagulant of choice is sodium heparin because small amounts of this particular anti-clotting agent does not affect the pH of the blood.

Indications

Arterial blood gas analysis is routinely ordered for patients who are receiving oxygen therapy or mechanical ventilation. In addition, an analysis may be indicated by the presence of an abnormal breathing pattern or increased work of breathing. Except in emergency cases, collection of the sample should be delayed at least 30 minutes following any changes in the ventilatory treatment or in the concentration of oxygen being delivered. This assures that the blood gas values have had an opportunity to stabilize. When collecting a sample for blood gas analysis, it is essential that ventilator settings and precise oxygen concentration or liter flow be recorded.

Potential Hazards

Arterial puncture, if done improperly, can result in a blood clot, arterial spasm, or hematoma at the puncture site. Sometimes, even when correct technique is used, arterial damage can occur. Damage to the artery itself poses a significant risk to the patient because the flow of blood to tissue distal to the puncture site could be partially or totally restricted. For this reason, the presence of collateral circulation is an important consideration when selecting a puncture site. Hematoma can normally be prevented by applying pressure to the site after puncture until the bleeding has completely subsided.

The most common sites for arterial blood sampling are the radial, brachial, and femoral arteries. Of these locations, the radial artery is generally preferred because it is more readily accessible and collateral circulation is provided by the ulnar artery.

The Allen test should always be performed prior to puncture of the radial artery to assess the adequacy of collateral circulation to the hand through the ulnar artery. A lack of collateral circulation indicates that there may be an occlusion of the ulnar artery. In such cases, the Allen test should be repeated on the opposite arm. If occlusion is detected in either or both of the ulnar arteries, the physician should be notified.

Procedure for Arterial Blood Sampling

It is recommended that arterial blood sampling be performed according to the following procedure:

A. *Check Order.* Verify the physician's order as follows:

1. Compare the requisition with the physician's order to ensure that no discrepancies exist.

2. If any part of the order is unfamiliar, question its accuracy.

B. *Assure Stabilization.* Except in an emergency situation, make certain that at least 30 minutes have elapsed since:

- Any change in the concentration of oxygen being delivered
- Any change in the oxygen therapy device being used
- Any interruption in the oxygen therapy delivered
- Any change in mechanical ventilator settings
- The administration of a respiratory therapy treatment

C. *Maintain Asepsis.* While performing the remainder of this procedure, you are expected to maintain aseptic conditions according to the procedures described in **SSE 1.2.** This includes the use of universal precautions and handwashing. Gloves must be worn during the actual puncture and anytime when the blood sample is being handled. Hands should be washed:

- Before obtaining equipment
- Following performance of step *L. Conclude Procedure*
- Anytime during the procedure that contamination is suspected.

D. *Obtain Equipment.* Make certain that you have the following equipment and supplies available:

- Gloves
- 3-5 cc heparinized syringe
- 1 inch, 23-25 gauge, beveled needle
- 1 1/2 inch, 21 gauge, beveled needle
- Syringe cap
- Betadine swab
- Alcohol swab
- Ice water bath
- Bandaid (optional)

E. *Assemble Equipment.* Prepare the equipment for use as follows:

1. Attach the capped needle to the syringe. (The 1 inch needle is usually used for a radial puncture. The 1 1\2 inch needle is used for brachial or femoral punctures).

2. Heparinize the syringe according to the manufacturer's instructions.

F. ***Confirm Patient.*** Ensure that the procedure is performed on the correct patient as follows:

1. Match the information on the order with the following:

   • Room number
   • Name on the door or bed
   • Name on the wristband

2. Greet the patient by name (in a questioning manner if unknown).

3. Resolve any discrepancies in the patient identification information by conferring with the nursing staff.

G. ***Inform Patient.*** Interact with the patient as follows:

1. Introduce yourself by name and department (if not already acquainted).

2. Tell the patient what procedure is to be performed.

3. Explain the procedure by describing:

   • Why it is to be performed
   • How it will be performed
   • What the patient is expected to do
   • What you will be doing
   • How frequently it will be performed

H. ***Perform Allen Test.*** Perform the following tasks:

1. Palpate the radial and ulnar pulses.

2. Instruct the patient to open and close the hand into a tight fist several times.

3. Apply sufficient pressure to the radial and ulnar arteries to cause the palm of the hand to blanch as it opens and closes.

4. Instruct the patient to relax the hand.

5. Release pressure over the ulnar artery.

6. If color does not return to the hand, repeat the above steps on the other arm.

7. If collateral circulation is not present in either hand, inform the evaluator.

I. **Implement Procedure.** Perform the following tasks:

1. Swab the selected puncture site with betadine.

2. While palpating the pulse with the opposite hand, slowly insert the needle into the artery until arterial blood is visualized in the hub of the syringe (bevel of needle facing up and needle entering the artery at a 45 to 60 degree angle).

3. Once the artery is punctured, allow arterial pressure to fill the syringe.

4. When approximately 1 to 2 cc of arterial blood are obtained, slowly remove the needle.

5. Immediately apply pressure over the puncture site with the sterile gauze pad until bleeding stops. (Apply pressure for at least 5 minutes.)

6. While applying pressure to the site, carefully remove any air bubbles from the syringe and briskly rotate the syringe in the hand to dissolve and mix the heparin.

7. Replace the protective covering on the needle before removing from syringe. Be especially careful to avoid needle sticks by using the hands free technique.

8. Being careful to prevent air bubbles from entering, quickly cap the syringe and place it in the ice water bath.

9. Dispose of the capped needle in the appropriate hazardous materials receptacle.

J. **Monitor Patient.** Determine the patient's response to the therapy as follows:

1. Determine the pulse rate. (Count for at least one minute).

2. Determine the respiratory rate. (Count for at least one minute).

3. Note any abnormalities in the patient's appearance or behavior.

K. **Record data.** Record the following data on the laboratory data form and on patient chart as required:

• Patient name
• Room number
• Pulse rate

- Respiratory rate
- Oxygen concentration or liter flow and delivery device
- Ventilator settings (as applicable)
- Puncture site
- Any adverse patient reactions
- Amount of time pressure was applied to site

L.   ***Conclude Procedure.***   Complete the following tasks:

1. Place the patient in a comfortable position.

2. Assure that the call bell and bedside table are within the patient's reach.

3. Ask if the patient has any needs.

4. Answer any questions as effectively as possible.

5. Inspect the puncture site to ensure that the bleeding has stopped.

6. Apply a bandaid to the site (optional).

M.   ***Report Observations.***   Report the following information:

1. Report any significant adverse changes in the patient's condition to the nurse or physician.

2. Following the procedure, inform the appropriate personnel of:

   - Patient requests
   - Patient complaints
   - Unexpressed patient needs

3. Following the procedure, report to the nurse or physician:

   - Any noncritical adverse reactions to the therapy
   - Other pertinent observations of the patient's condition

N.   ***Dispense Sample.***   Send the blood sample and the completed data form to the appropriate laboratory for analysis.

Ancillary Procedure 6.3
Pulse Oximetry

The assessment of oxygenation by sampling arterial blood is an invasive process that can result in damage to the artery. Because of this potential danger, noninvasive methods of assessing oxygenation have been developed. Pulse oximetry is a common method of noninvasive measurement of oxygen levels in the blood.

Pulse oximetry provides an indirect measurement of oxygen saturation in the blood. By directing a light source through transparent tissue of the body (i.e., finger or earlobe) the amount of oxygen carried by the hemoglobin in the blood (oxygen saturation) can be indirectly measured. The measurement is dependent upon the availability of an adequate supply of blood at the site of the oximeter probe. As long as perfusion to the site is adequate, however, the oxygen saturation level reported by the oximeter will be accurate. Nearly all oximeters are equipped with an alarm that will sound to indicate when perfusion to the site is inadequate.

This method of oxygen monitoring eliminates the pain and potential hazards associated with arterial puncture. Because of its accuracy and the elimination of dangerous side effects, pulse oximeter has become increasingly popular in the assessment of oxygenation. It should be noted, however, that oximetry does not replace arterial blood gas sampling because carbon dioxide levels cannot be measured with an oximeter.

Indications

Pulse oximetry is ordered to assess the oxygenation of patients receiving oxygen therapy or mechanical ventilation. Ordinarily, an initial determination of oxygenation should be performed by means of a direct measurement of arterial blood gases. Once the patient's overall ventilation has been assessed, oximetry can be performed on an ongoing basis to assess the continuing need for oxygen.

Oximetry can be performed intermittently or on a continuous basis. For the stable patient on oxygen therapy, intermittent oximetry can be performed to assess patient progress. For the unstable patient, however, oximetry should be performed continuously to provide immediate information whenever there is an increase in the patient's oxygen requirements.

Potential Hazards

The non-invasive nature of pulse oximetry makes it essentially hazard-free. There are times when a patient could be at risk, however, because of the limitations of oximetry in providing an accurate assessment of the level of oxygenation. It was noted that perfusion to the site of the oximetry probe will greatly affect accuracy of results. Whenever there is any reason to doubt the accuracy of an oximetry reading, arterial blood gases should be obtained for verification of oxygen levels.

Procedure for Performing Pulse Oximetry

It is recommended that pulse oximetry be performed according to the following procedure:

A. **Check Order.** Verify the physician's order as follows:

1. Compare the requisition with the physician's order to ensure that no discrepancies exist.

2. If any part of the order is unfamiliar, question its accuracy.

B. **Assure Stabilization.** Except in an emergency situation, make certain that at least 30 minutes have elapsed since:

- Any change in the concentration of oxygen being delivered
- Any change in the oxygen therapy device being used
- Any interruption in the oxygen therapy delivered
- Any change in mechanical ventilator settings
- The administration of a respiratory therapy treatment

C. **Maintain Asepsis.** While performing the remainder of this procedure, you are expected to maintain aseptic conditions according to the procedures described in **SSE 1.2**. This includes the use of universal precautions and handwashing. Hands should be washed:

- Before obtaining equipment
- Following performance of step **L. Conclude Procedure**
- Anytime during the procedure that contamination is suspected

D. **Obtain Equipment.** Collect the following equipment and supplies:

- Oximeter
- Oximeter probe
- Alcohol swab

E. *Assemble Equipment.* Prepare the equipment for use as follows:

1. Calibrate the oximeter according to the manufacturer's instructions.

2. Attach the proper probe to the oximeter.

F. *Confirm Patient.* Ensure that the procedure is performed on the correct patient as follows:

1. Match the information on the order with the following:

   • Room number
   • Name on the door or bed
   • Name on the wristband

2. Greet the patient by name (in a questioning manner if unknown).

3. Resolve any discrepancies in the patient identification information by conferring with the nursing staff.

G. *Inform Patient.* Interact with the patient as follows:

1. Introduce yourself by name and department (if not already acquainted).

2. Tell the patient what procedure is to be performed.

3. Explain the procedure by describing:

   • Why it is to be performed
   • How it will be performed
   • What the patient is expected to do
   • What you will be doing
   • How frequently it will be performed

H. *Assess Perfusion to Site.* Perform the following tasks:

1. If a finger probe is being used, select a finger that shows evidence of good perfusion and is free of fingernail polish. If there is poor perfusion to both hands, use an ear probe.

2. If an ear probe is used, swab the earlobe with alcohol to remove any oils. Gently rub the earlobe between the thumb and finger for sixty seconds to enhance perfusion.

I. ***Implement Procedure.*** Perform the following tasks:

1. Place the probe on the finger or earlobe and obtain the pulse and oxygen saturation results from the oximeter.

2. If oximetry is to be continuous, secure the probe as necessary to ensure that it does not become displaced.

3. If oximetry is to be continuous, set oximetry alarms according to the physician's order.

J. ***Monitor Patient.*** Determine the patient's response to the therapy as follows:

1. Determine the pulse rate. (Count for at least one minute).

2. Compare the patient's pulse rate at the wrist to the value given by the oximeter to verify the accuracy of the results.

3. Determine the respiratory rate. (Count for at least one minute).

4. Note any abnormalities in the patient's appearance or behavior.

K. ***Record data.*** Record the following data on the patient's chart as required:

- Patient's name
- Room number
- Pulse rate
- Respiratory rate
- Oxygen saturation results
- Oxygen concentration or liter flow and delivery device
- Ventilator settings (as applicable)
- Any adverse patient reactions

L. ***Conclude Procedure.*** Complete the following tasks:

1. Place the patient in a comfortable position.

2. Assure that the call bell and bedside table are within the patient's reach.

3. Ask if the patient has any needs.

4. Answer any questions as effectively as possible.

Notes

M. ***Report Observations.*** Report the following information:

1. Report any significant adverse changes in the patient's condition to the nurse or physician.

2. Following the procedure, inform the appropriate personnel of:

   • Patient requests
   • Patient complaints
   • Unexpressed patient needs

3. Following the procedure, report to the nurse or physician:

   • Any non-critical adverse reactions to the therapy
   • Other pertinent observations of the patient's condition

Ancillary Procedure 6.4
Capnography

Capnography is a method for obtaining an indirect measurement of carbon dioxide levels in the body. The procedure provides a noninvasive alternative to arterial puncture. A capnograph is a device that measures the actual amount of carbon dioxide in exhaled gases. The value obtained is termed end-tidal CO_2 ($ETCO_2$). End-tidal CO_2 correlates directly with the amount of carbon dioxide in arterial blood. The normal value obtained for the end-tidal CO_2 will be somewhat lower than the PCO_2, but the values should be parallel to each other giving a general indication of the level of arterial CO_2.

End-tidal CO_2 is measured continuously. It is difficult to monitor unless the patient is intubated and mechanically ventilated. Arterial blood gases should be obtained at the time of the initial capnograph reading to verify its accuracy. Once the accuracy of the capnograph has been established, the $ETCO_2$ serves as a good indicator of arterial CO_2, but it gives no information regarding the oxygen level. A pulse oximeter can be used in conjunction with the $ETCO_2$ monitor to reflect both O_2 and CO_2 levels.

Indications

Capnography is useful for monitoring CO_2 levels on a continuous basis. The procedure is indicated when weaning a patient from mechanical ventilation or anytime carbon dioxide levels are unstable during mechanical ventilation. Carbon dioxide monitoring is commonly used with head injury patients when it is important that CO_2 levels are kept low.

Potential Hazards

Because capnography is noninvasive, there are relatively few physical hazards that accompany the procedure. The primary concern when using the procedure to monitor CO_2 levels is the accuracy of the values obtained. If the $ETCO_2$ values are not verified periodically by comparing them to the values obtained from a direct analysis of arterial blood gases, a dangerous situation could be created by relying on inaccurate values. When in doubt about the accuracy of the capnograph, notify the nurse or physician immediately.

Procedure for Capnography

It is recommended that capnography be performed according to the following procedure:

A.   ***Check Order.*** Verify the physician's order as follows:

   1.   Compare the requisition with the physician's order to ensure that no discrepancies exist.

   2.   If any part of the order is unfamiliar, question its accuracy.

B.   ***Maintain Asepsis.*** While performing the remainder of this procedure, you are expected to maintain aseptic conditions according to the procedures described in **SSE 1.2**. This includes the use of universal precautions and handwashing. Hands should be washed:

   • Before obtaining equipment
   • Following performance of step ***J. Conclude Procedure***
   • Anytime during the procedure that contamination is suspected

C.   ***Obtain Equipment.*** Collect the following equipment and supplies:

   • Capnograph
   • CO_2 transducer
   • Calibration gas

D.   ***Assemble Equipment.*** Calibrate the capnograph according to the manufacturer's instructions.

E.   ***Confirm Patient.*** Ensure that the procedure is performed on the correct patient as follows:

   1.   Match the information on the order with the following:

      • Room number
      • Name on the door or bed
      • Name on the wristband

   2.   Greet the patient by name (in a questioning manner if unknown).

   3.   Resolve any discrepancies in the patient identification information by conferring with the nursing staff.

F. *Inform Patient.* Interact with the patient as follows:

1. Introduce yourself by name and department (if not already acquainted).

2. Tell the patient what procedure is to be performed.

3. Explain the procedure by describing:

    • Why it is to be performed
    • How it will be performed
    • What the patient is expected to do
    • What you will be doing
    • How frequently it will be performed

G. *Implement Procedure.* Perform the following tasks:

1. Place the CO_2 transducer within the ventilator circuit close to the airway adaptor.

2. Secure the transducer as necessary to ensure that it does not become displaced or pull on the endotracheal tube.

3. Set the capnograph alarms according to the physician's order.

4. Allow the capnograph to stabilize and verify the results by comparing them to the arterial blood gas results.

H. *Monitor Patient.* Determine the patient's response to the therapy as follows:

1. Determine the pulse rate. (Count for at least one minute).

2. Determine the respiratory rate. (Count for at least one minute).

3. Note any abnormalities in the patient's appearance or behavior.

I. *Record data.* Record the following data on the patient's chart as required:

    • Patient name
    • Room number
    • Pulse rate
    • Respiratory rate
    • Capnography results
    • Ventilator settings
    • Any adverse patient reactions

Notes

J. *Conclude Procedure.* Complete the following tasks:

1. Place the patient in a comfortable position.

2. Assure that the call bell and bedside table are within the patient's reach.

3. Ask if the patient has any needs.

4. Answer any questions as effectively as possible.

K. *Report Observations.* Report the following information:

1. Report any significant adverse changes in the patient's condition to the nurse or physician.

2. Following the procedure, inform the appropriate personnel of:

   • Patient requests
   • Patient complaints
   • Unexpressed patient needs

3. Following the procedure, report to the nurse or physician:

   • Any non-critical adverse reactions to the therapy
   • Other pertinent observations of the patient's condition

Ancillary Procedure 6.5
Transcutaneous Monitoring

Transcutaneous monitoring is a noninvasive method for the indirect assessment of arterial blood gas levels. This method involves the placement of a heated probe on the skin and the measurement of the blood gas levels in the transcutaneous tissue at the point of placement. The value obtained by this method correlates directly with the blood gas levels in the arteries. As with all non invasive monitors, an initial blood gas value should be obtained from a sample of arterial blood to verify accuracy of the monitor.

Indications

A transcutaneous monitor provides a measure of blood gas values on a continuous basis. Most transcutaneous monitors can measure both oxygen and carbon dioxide levels in circulating blood, but some are designed to measure only oxygen. The use of a transcutaneous monitor is indicated for patients with unstable blood gases. Typically, a patient on mechanical ventilation or with pending respiratory failure would benefit from continuous monitoring of oxygen and/or carbon dioxide levels. In addition, transcutaneous monitor are often used with premature infants who can have rapid changes in respiratory status.

Potential Hazards

Transcutaneous monitors use a heated probe to measure blood gas values through the skin. There is a danger of tissue damage if the probe temperature is too hot or if the probe remains in one place too long. For this reason, close attention must be paid to the manufacturer's guidelines for controlling the temperature of the probe and for changing its placement on the skin.

As with all monitors that measure blood gas values indirectly, the accuracy of the transcutaneous monitor should be frequently assessed by comparing the values obtained with the monitor to those obtained by analyzing a sample of arterial blood. If a discrepancy exists in the values obtained by the two different methods, the nurse or physician should be consulted immediately.

Procedure for Transcutaneous Monitoring

It is recommended that transcutaneous monitoring be performed according to the following procedure:

A. Check Order. Verify the physician's order as follows:

    1. Compare the requisition with the physician's order to ensure that no discrepancies exist.

    2. If any part of the order is unfamiliar, question its accuracy.

B. Maintain Asepsis. While performing the remainder of this procedure, you are expected to maintain aseptic conditions according to the procedures described in **SSE 1.2**. This includes the use of universal precautions and handwashing. Hands should be washed:

    • Before obtaining equipment
    • Following performance of step *J. Conclude Procedure*
    • Anytime during the procedure that contamination is suspected

C. Obtain Equipment. Collect the following equipment and supplies:

    • Transcutaneous Monitor
    • Calibration gas (for CO_2 monitoring only)
    • Electrode calibration kit
    • Oxygen and carbon dioxide electrodes (as applicable)
    • Alcohol swab
    • Electrode application ring
    • Electrode placement solution

D. Assemble Equipment. Calibrate the transcutaneous monitor according to the manufacturer's instructions.

E. Confirm Patient. Ensure that the procedure is performed on the correct patient as follows:

    1. Match the information on the order with the following:

        • Room number
        • Name on the door or bed
        • Name on the wristband

    2. Greet the patient by name (in a questioning manner if unknown).

    3. Resolve any discrepancies in the patient identification information by conferring with the nursing staff.

F. **Inform Patient.** Interact with the patient as follows:

1. Introduce yourself by name and department (if not already acquainted).

2. Tell the patient what procedure is to be performed.

3. Explain the procedure by describing:

    • Why it is to be performed
    • How it will be performed
    • What the patient is expected to do
    • What you will be doing
    • How frequently it will be performed

G. **Implement Procedure.** Perform the following tasks:

1. After calibrating the electrode and setting the monitor according to manufacturer's guidelines, select a fleshy area on the patient's upper chest wall for placement of the electrode.

2. Swab the skin area selected with alcohol to remove any oils. Allow the skin to dry completely.

3. Adhere the placement ring to the electrode and remove the backing so that the electrode is surrounded by a sticky adhesive ring.

4. Place a small drop of electrode placement solution in the center of the electrode.

5. Without spilling the drop of solution, place the electrode firmly against the skin making certain that the surrounding adhesive is secured to the skin.

6. Allow the monitor to stabilize and compare the values obtained to the most recent arterial blood gas values. If a discrepancy exists, notify the nurse or physician immediately.

H. **Monitor Patient.** Determine the patient's response to the therapy as follows:

1. Determine the pulse rate. (Count for at least one minute).

2. Determine the respiratory rate. (Count for at least one minute).

3. Note any abnormalities in the patient's appearance or behavior.

I. **Record data.** Record the following data on the patient's chart as required:

- Patient name
- Room number
- Pulse rate
- Respiratory rate
- Transcutaneous blood gas values
- Placement site of electrode
- Electrode temperature
- Ventilator settings
- Any adverse patient reactions

J. **Conclude Procedure.** Complete the following tasks:

1. Place the patient in a comfortable position.

2. Assure that the call bell and bedside table are within the patient's reach.

3. Ask if the patient has any needs.

4. Answer any questions as effectively as possible.

K. **Report Observations.** Report the following information:

1. Report any significant adverse changes in the patient's condition to the nurse or physician.

2. Following the procedure, inform the appropriate personnel of:

   - Patient requests
   - Patient complaints
   - Unexpressed patient needs

3. Following the procedure, report to the nurse or physician:

   - Any non-critical adverse reactions to the procedure
   - Other pertinent observations of the patient's condition

Evaluation of Advanced Assessment Procedures

The following definitions are provided for use whenever the respective Advanced Assessment Procedures are evaluated. In order for performance of the procesedures to be considered acceptable, all Essential Tasks are to be performed according to the eccompanying Evaluation Criteria. Any deviation from the following task sequence or criteria must be approved by the evaluator.

APE 6.1 Ventilatory Assessment		
Performance	**Essential Tasks**	**Evaluation Criteria**
A. Maintain Asepsis	See SSE 1.2	See SSE 1.2
B. Prepare Equipment	1. Obtains and assembles: • Spirometer and Patient attachment • Negative pressure manometer and patient attachment	a. Correct equipment used for procedure b. Equipment functioned properly after assembly
C. Confirm Patient	See SSE 3.3	See SSE 3.3
D. Inform Patient	See SSE 4.1	See SSE 4.1
E. Demonstrate FVC, V_T and $\dot{V}_E$ Procedures	1. Shows patient how to: • Use attachment • Breathe normally • Inhale maximally • Exhale rapidly and completely 2. Describes procedure while demonstrating	a. Demonstrated correctly b. Did not contaminate attachment a. Described accurately b. Effort made to assure patient understanding

APE 6.1
Ventilatory Assessment (continued)

Performance	Essential Tasks	Evaluation Criteria
F. Implement FVC, V_T and $\dot{V}_E$ Procedures	1. Positions patient	a. Placed in upright position (45-90°)
	2. Attaches equipment to patient	a. Attachment device correctly positioned b. Noseclip firmly attached (when needed)
	3. Directs patient actions	a. Patient encouraged to exert maximum effor for FVC b. Procedure repeated (at least 3 times) with adequate rest between
	4. Determines assessment results	a. All FVC, V_T and $\dot{V}_E$ data recorded b. Average V_T calculated properly c. Best FVC selected
G. Demonstrate MIP Procedure	1. Shows patient how to: • Use attachment • Exhale maximally • Inhale maximally	a. Demonstrated correctly b. Did not contaminate attachment
	2. Describes procedure while demonstrating patient understanding	a. Described accurately b. Effort made to assure
H. Implement MIP Procedure	1. Attaches equipment to patient	a. Attachment device correctly positioned b. Noseclip firmly attached (when needed)
	2. Directs patient actions	a. Patient encouraged to exert maximum effort to MIP b. Procedure repeated (at least three times) with adequate rests between
	3. Determines assessment results	a. All MIP data recorded b. Best MIP selected
I. Conclude Procedure	1. Restores room to original condition	a. Equipment removed from room or covered and moved to suitable location within room b. Call bell and bedside table positioned within patient's reach

APE 6.1		
Ventilatory Assessment (continued)		
Performance	**Essential Tasks**	**Evaluation Criteria**
I. Conclude Procedure (continued)	2. Tends to patient needs	a. Comfortable position assured b. Patient asked regarding other needs c. Patient questions answered effectively
J. Record	See SSE 3.4	See SSE 3.4
K. Report Observations	See SSE 4.3	See SSE 4.3

APE 6.2
Arterial Blood Sampling

Performance	Essential Tasks	Evaluation Criteria
A. Check Order	See SSE 3.1	See SSE 3.1
B. Assure Stabilization	1. Confirms correct oxygen delivery or ventilator settings	a. Prescribed oxygen concentration assured b. Prescribed delivery device assured c. Prescribed ventilator settings assured
	2. Ensures adequate stabilization	a. Sample not collected unless patient was stabilized for at least 30 minutes
C. Maintain Asepsis	See SSE 1.2	See SSE 1.2
D. Obtain Equipment	1. Obtains the following equipment and supplies: • Gloves • Heparinized syringe • Correct needle size • Syringe cap • Betadine swab • Alcohol swab • Ice water bath • Bandaid (optional)	a. Correct equipment obtained
E. Assemble Equipment	1. Prepares equipment as follows: • Attaches needle to syringe • Heparinzes syringe.	a. Assembled according to SOP
F. Confirm Patient	See SSE 3.3	See SSE 3.3
G. Inform Patient	See SSE 4.1	See SSE 4.1

APE 6.2
Arterial Blood Sampling (continued)

Performance	Essential Tasks	Evaluation Criteria
H. Perform Allen Test	1. Palpates arteries	a. Correctly located: • Radial artery • Ulnar artery
	2. Instructs patient to make fist	a. Clean and accurate instructions provided b. Instructions repeated as necessary to obtain patient compliance
	3. Applies pressure over arteries	a. Hand blanched
	4. Instructs patient to relax hand	a. Clean and accurate instructions provided b. Instruction repeated as necessary to obtain patient compliance
	5. Completes Allen test	a. Pressure over ulnar artery released b. Pressure still applied over radial artery c. Results interpreted correctly
	6. Repeats steps on other hand if artery occluded	a. Procedure repeated correctly b. Physician notified if one or both ulnar arteries occluded
I. Implement Procedure	1. Swabs puncture site	a. Betadine used b. Correct area swabbed c. Area swabbed thoroughly
	2. Inserts needle	a. Pulse palpated with non-dominant hand b. Needle inserted; • In artery • At 45-60° angle • Bevel of needle up
	3. Collects blood sample	a. Adequate sample for blood gas analyzer obtained
	4. Removes needle	a. Removed slowly
	5. Applies pressure over artery	a. Adequate pressure applied to stop bleeding b. Pressure applied for 5 minutes or longer if necessary to stop bleeding

APE 6.2 Arterial Blood Sampling (continued)		
Performance	**Essential Tasks**	**Evaluation Criteria**
I. Implement Procedure (continued)	6. Places syringe in ice	a. Air bubbles removed b. Syringe capped
J. Monitor Patient	1. Determines: • Pulse rate • Respiratory rate 2. Observes: • Patient appearance • Patient behavior	a. Counted for at lease one (1) minute a. Any abnormalities identified
K. Record Data	1. Records the following: • Patient's name • Room number • Pulse rate • Respiratory rate • Oxygen concentration or liter flow • Oxygen delivery device • Puncture site • ventilator settings (as applicable)	a. Data recorded accurately
L. Conclude Procedure	1. Replace call bell and bedside table 2. Tends to patient needs 3. Rechecks puncture site at least 5-10 minutes after procedure	a. Placed within patient's reach a. Comfortable position assured b. Patient asked regarding other needs c. Patient questions answered effectively a. Rechecked 5-10 minutes after procedure b. Inspected for hematoma c. Pressure reapplied if still bleeding
M. Report Observations	See SSE 4.3	See SSE 4.3

APE 6.2 Arterial Blood Sampling (continued)		
Performance	**Essential Tasks**	**Evaluation Criteria**
N. Dispense Sample	1. Sends blood sample to appropriate lab	a. Sample sent to appropriate lab
	2. Completes data form	a. Data from completed and sent to appropriate lab

	APE 6.3	
	Pulse Oximetry	
Performance	**Essential Tasks**	**Evaluation Criteria**
A. Check Order	See **SSE 3.1**	See **SSE 3.1**
B. Assure Stabilization	1. Confirms correct oxygen delivery or ventilator settings	a. Prescribed oxygen delivery percentage assured b. Prescribed delivery device assured c. Prescribed ventilator settings assured
	2. Ensures adequate stabilization	a. Measurement not taken unless patient stabilized for at least 30 minutes
C. Maintain Asepsis	See **SSE 1.2**	See **SSE 1.2**
D. Obtain Equipment	1. Obtains the following equipment: • Oximeter • Probe • Alcohol swab	a. Correct equipment obtained
E. Assemble Equipment	1. Prepares equipment as follows: • Calibrates oximeter • Attaches probe to oximeter	a. Assembled according to **SOP**
F. Confirm Patient	See **SSE 3.3**	See **SSE 3.3**
G. Inform Patient	See **SSE 4.1**	See **SSE 4.1**
H. Assess Perfusion to Site	1. Assess finger for: • Good perfusion • Nail polish	a. Finger not used if perfusion poor or nailpolish present
	2. Prepares ear: swabs with alcohol rubs for 60 seconds	a. Earlobe properly prepared

APE 6.3
Pulse Oximetry (continued)

Performance	Essential Tasks	Evaluation Criteria
I. Implement Procedure	1. Places probe on finger or ear	a. Correctly positions probe
	2. Secures probe if oximetry is continuous	a. Probe properly secured
	3. Sets alarms if oximetry is continuous	a. Alarms set according to physcican order
J. Monitor Patient	1. Determines: • Pulse rate • Respirations	a. Counted for at least one (1) minute
	2. Compares pulse rate to oximeter	a. Matches pulse rate
	3. Observes: • Patient appearance • Patient behavior	a. Any abnormalities identified
K. Record Data	1. Records the following: • Patient's name • Room number • Pulse rate • Respiratory rate • Oxygen concentration or liter flow • Oxygen delivery device • Probe site • Ventilator settings (as applicable)	a. Data recorded accurately
L. Conclude Procedure	1. Replaces call bell and bedside table	a. Placed within patient's reach
	2. Tends to patient needs	a. Comfortable position assured b. Patient asked regarding other needs c. Patient questions answered effectively
M. Report Observations	See SSE 4.3	See SSE 4.3

APE 6.4 Capnography		
Performance	**Essential Tasks**	**Evaluation Critieria**
A. Check Order	See SSE 3.1	See SSE 3.1
B. Maintain Asepsis	See SSE 1.2	See SSE 1.2
C. Obtain Equipment	1. Obtains the following equipment. • Capnograph • CO_2 Transducer • Calibration Gas	a. Correct equipment obtained
D. Assemble Equipment	1. Prepares equipment as follows: • Calibrates according to manufacturer guidelines	a. Assembled and calibrated according to SOP
E. Confirm Patient	See SSE 3.3	See SSE 3.3
F. Inform Patient	See SSE 4.1	See SSE 4.1
G. Implement Patient	1. Places transducer in circuit close to airway 2. Secures transducer transducer 3. Sets alarms 4. Allows to stabilize	a. Transducer correctly placed a. Transducer secrued properly a. Alarms set a. Unit stabilized
H. Monitor Patient	1. Determines: • Pulse rate • Respirations 2. Observes: • Patient appearance • Patient behavior	a. Counted for at least one (1) minute a. Any abnormalities identified

	APE 6.4	
	Capnography (continued)	
Performace	**Essential Tasks**	**Evaluation Criteria**
I. Record Data	1. Records the following: • Patient's name • Room number • Pulse rate • Respiratory rate • Oxygen delivery device • Ventilators settings (as applicable)	a. Data recorded accurately
J. Conclude Procedure	1. Replaces call bell and bedside table	a. Places within patient's reach
	2. Tends to patient needs	a. Comfortable position assured b. Patient asked regarding other needs c. Patient's questions answered effectively
K. Report Observations	See **SSE 4.3**	See **SSE 4.3**

APE 6.5 Transcutaneous Monitoring		
Performance	**Essential Tasks**	**Evaluation Criteria**
A. Check Order	See SSE 3.1	See SSE 3.1
B. Maintain Asepsis	See SSE 1.2	See SSE 1.2
C. Obtain Equipment	1. Obtains the following equipment: • Monitor • Electorde calibration kit • Calibration Gas (CO_2 monitoring only) • O_2 and/or CO_2 electrodes • Alcohol swab • Electrode application ring • Electrode placement solution	a. Correct equipment obtained
D. Assemble Equipment	1. Prepares equipment as follows • Calibrates according to manufacturer guidelines	a. Assembled and calibrated according to SOP
E. Confirm Patient	See SSE 3.3	See SSE 3.3
F. Inform Patient	See SSE 4.1	See SSE 4.1
G. Implement Procedure	1. Selects fleshy area for electrode placement	a. Site selected appropriately
	2. Swabs site with alcohol	a. Site cleaned properly
	3. Adheres electrode ring	a. Ring secured properly
	4. Places drop of electrode fluid	a. Fluid placed properly
	5. Places electrode	a. Electrode placed properly
	6. Allows monitor to stabilize	a. Units allowed to stabilize

APE 6.5		
Transcutaneous Monitoring (continued)		
Performance	**Essential Tasks**	**Evaluation Criteria**
H. Monitor Patient	1. Determines: • Pulse rate • Respirations 2. Observes: • Patient appearance • Patient behavior	a. Counted for at least one (1) minute a. Any abnormalities identified
I. Record Data	1. Recordes the following: • Patient's name • Room number • Pulse rate • Respiratory rate • Oxygen delivery device • Ventilator settings (as applicable)	a. Data recorded accurately
J. Conclude Procedure	1. Replaces call bell and bedside table 2. Tends to patient needs	a. Places within patient's reach a. Comfortable position assured b. Patient asked regarding other needs c. Patient's questions answered effectively
K. Report Observations	See SSE 4.3	See SSE 4.3

Module 7.0

Breathing Exercises

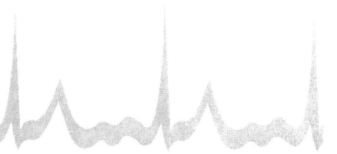

Certain patients need to increase the efficiency of the breathing process because they do not take full advantage of proper breathing mechanics. In many instances, their situation is further complicated by the physical and emotional stress of chronic pulmonary disease. Paraplegic and quadriplegic patients often require special assistance with coughing in order to remove secretions from their airways. It is often possible for these individuals to improve their breathing efficiency by learning and practicing proper breathing methods. Training in the methods of diaphragmatic breathing, pursed lip breathing, and cough assist is commonly provided to such patients. These three methods are described in the present module.

Objectives

Upon completion of this module, you will be able to:

1. Identify patients who could benefit from breathing exercises.

2. Demonstrate and teach a patient to employ the technique of diaphragmatic breathing.

3. Demonstrate and teach a patient to employ the technique of pursed lip breathing.

4. Demonstrate and teach a patient to employ the technique of cough assist.

Breathing is a natural body process controlled by the autonomic nervous system. In the normal individual, the expiratory phase is approximately one and one-half times as long as the inspiratory phase. The inspiratory phase is shorter because inspiration is an active process characterized by contraction of respiratory muscles, while expiration occurs passively as these muscles relax.

Any condition that alters the normal breathing process increases the work of breathing. This includes temporary emotional states resulting from factors such as fear, pain, or excitement and more permanent conditions associated with pulmonary disease or muscle paralysis. Whenever the work of breathing is increased by such conditions, training to increase breathing efficiency is indicated. The three breathing methods for which training is most commonly provided are diaphragmatic breathing, breathing with pursed lips, and cough assist.

Training in proper breathing technique usually must include considerations for patient motivation. Because the patient has been breathing in a certain "style" for all of his or her life, it may be necessary to provide a convincing rationale in order to gain compliance. The rationale might include such factors as decreasing shortness of breath, increasing exercise tolerance, removal of secretions, prevention of infection, and reducing the work of breathing. To enhance patient cooperation, it is best to introduce training in breathing procedures when the patient is experiencing little or no respiratory difficulty.

Ancillary Procedure 7.1
Diaphragmatic Breathing

The inspiratory phase of the breathing cycle results from contraction of the respiratory muscles. The most efficient of these muscles is the diaphragm. Because the human body tends to function in an efficient manner, the majority of the inspiratory effort is normally provided by the diaphragm. Any condition that increases reliance upon the intercostal and accessory muscles tends to reduce breathing efficiency.

Factors such as poor posture and pulmonary disorders that cause shortness of breath often increase dependence on the intercostal and accessory muscles. Reliance upon these muscles is further increased by COPD because greater than normal lung volumes at end-expiration prevent the diaphragm from returning to its normal resting level. Paraplegics and quadriplegics often lose the use of their accessory muscles and must rely completely upon the diaphragm in order to breathe. Regardless of the reason for poor breathing technique, greater use of the diaphragm for inspiration will improve breathing efficiency.

More efficient breathing habits can be encouraged by training a patient to perform diaphragmatic breathing exercises. Such training may be difficult because of insufficient motivation on the part of the patient. In addition, the patient may become reluctant due to an increased work of breathing during early stages of the training. Such an increase in the effort required for breathing will be experienced until the diaphragm regains the strength lost as a result of reduced usage.

Indications

Training in the procedure of diaphragmatic breathing is most frequently provided as a part of pulmonary rehabilitation. In addition, the training often accompanies lung expansion therapy and aerosol administration. During IPPB and incentive spirometry, breathing diaphragmatically improves alveolar ventilation by increasing the depth of breathing. In the same way, it tends to improve particle deposition during aerosol therapy. In general, any obvious use of accessory muscles by a patient is an indication that diaphragmatic breathing exercises may be beneficial.

Procedure for Teaching Diaphragmatic Breathing

Whenever a need for increased use of diaphragmatic breathing is observed, instruct the patient as follows:

A. ***Demonstrate Procedure.*** Describe and demonstrate the following:

   1. Procedure for diaphragmatic breathing.

   2. Instruct the patient to watch while you:

      a. Place one hand on your abdomen.
      b. Move your abdomen out during slow inspiration.
      c. Move your abdomen in during slow expiration.

B. ***Position Patient.*** Place the patient in one of the following positions:

   • Supine with the knees flexed
   • Sitting on the side of the bed with the feet dangling
   • Standing up

C. ***Coach Patient.*** Coach the patient in the following manner:

   1. Place your hands or a weighted bag over the patient's abdomen.

   2. Instruct the patient to move the abdomen out during inspiration and in during expiration.

D. ***Complete Procedure.*** To complete the instruction for diaphragmatic breathing:

   1. Have the patient repeat the procedure until mastered.

   2. Provide maximal encouragement as the procedure is repeated.

   3. Encourage the patient to continue breathing diaphragmatically after the instruction is completed.

Ancillary Procedure 7.2
Pursed Lip Breathing

Patients with obstructive pulmonary disease tend to have an increased residual lung volume. The increased volume results from factors such as loss of elastic recoil of the lungs, early collapse of the small bronchioles during expiration, and increased expiratory air resistance due to turbulent flow. By breathing through pursed lips, the patient can increase the time spent in expiration by controlling and reducing expiratory flow rates. This technique tends to reduce the volume of gas remaining in the alveoli following expiration.

Indications

Pursed lip breathing is generally indicated whenever a COPD patient shows increased work of breathing. Because the patient is more likely to respond to this training when experiencing little or no breathing difficulty, it is frequently included as a part of pulmonary rehabilitation. Patient cooperation may be further enhanced by explaining the purpose of the breathing maneuver.

Procedure for Teaching Pursed Lip Breathing

Upon recognizing the need for pursed lip breathing, instruct the patient as follows:

A. *Demonstrate Procedure.* Instruct the patient to watch while you:

   1. Inhale slowly through your nose.

   2. Exhale slowly through pursed lips.

B. *Coach Patient.* Coach the patient to:

   1. Inhale slowly through the nose.

   2. Exhale slowly through pursed lips.

C.   *Complete Procedure.*   To complete the instruction for pursed lip breathing:

1. Have the patient repeat the procedure until mastered.

2. Provide maximal encouragement as the procedure is repeated.

3. Encourage the patient to continue exhaling through pursed lips after the instruction is completed.

Ancillary Procedure 7.3
Cough Assist

Quadriplegics and certain patients with muscle paralysis lose the use of the accessory muscles of ventilation and must rely solely upon the diaphragm for breathing. For this reason, such patients require special assistance with coughing and with the removal of secretions. By providing physical support to the diaphragm during the cough maneuver, an effective cough can be achieved and the retention of secretions can be prevented.

Indications

Cough assist is indicated whenever a muscle-impaired patient is having difficulty raising secretions. This means that such patients should be provided cough assist after every respiratory treatment and between treatments as needed. In most cases, a muscle-impaired patient will ask for help whenever cough assist is necessary. Cough assist does not have to be provided to patients who are able to cough effectively on their own.

Procedure for Providing Cough Assist

Whenever a muscle or neurologically-impaired patient has a need to learn the cough assist procedure, instruct the patient as follows:

A. *Demonstrate Procedure.* Describe and demonstrate the following:

   1. Procedure for cough assist.

   2. Instruct the patient to watch while you:

      a. Place both hands over your abdomen just beneath the rib cage.
      b. Move your abdomen out during a deep inspiration.
      c. Quickly and forcefully push your hands inward and upward beneath your rib cage during a forced cough effort.

B. *Assume Position.* Position the patient and yourself as follows:

1. Place the patient in a supine position.

2. Place your hands, one over the other, on the patient's abdomen just beneath the ribcage. (Place the heel of the lower hand in a position that allows you to push up toward the lungs.)

C. *Coach Patient.* Coach the patient in the following manner:

1. Instruct the patient to inhale deeply by moving the diaphragm out.

2. Instruct the patient to cough forcefully while you apply a quick and forceful upward thrust beneath the ribcage with the heels of the hands.

3. Assist the patient in removing any secretions. (Follow universal precautions.)

D. *Complete Procedure.* To complete the instruction for cough assist.

1. Repeat the procedure with the patient until mastered.

2. Provide maximal encouragement as the procedure is repeated.

3. Encourage the patient to request cough assist whenever difficulty in raising secretions occurs.

Evaluation of Breathing Exercise Procedures

The following definitions are provided for use whenever the respective Breathing Exercise Procedures are evaluated. In order for performance of the procedures to be considered acceptable, all Essential Tasks are to be performed according to the accompanying Evaluation Criteria. Any deviation from the following task sequence or criteria must be approved by the evaluator.

APE 7.1 Diaphragmatic Breathing		
Performance	**Essential Tasks**	**Evaluation Criteria**
A. Demonstrate Procedure	1. Instructs patient to observe demonstration 2. Performs the following: • Places hand on abdomen • Moves abdomen out while inhaling slowly • Moves abdomen in while exhaling slowly	a. Clear and accurate instructions provided a. Procedure demonstrated correctly
B. Position Patient	1. Places patient in one of the following positions: • Supine • Sitting, or • Standing	a. Appropriate position selected for patient condition: b. If supine, knees flexed; c. If sitting, feet dangling over side of the bed; d. If standing, upright with ⎿ ⏌k straight
C. Coach Patient	1. Places hands or weighted bag over abdomen 2. Instructs patient to: • Move abdomen out while inhaling • Move abdomen in while exhaling	a. Placed in correct position a. Clear and accurate instructions provided
D. Complete Procedure	1. Repeats breathing instructions	a. Previous step repeated until procedure mastered or patient tires

APE 7.1 Diaphragmatic Breathing (continued)		
Performance	**Essential Tasks**	**Evaluation Criteria**
D. Complete Procedure (continued)		b. Patient performance encouraged
	2. Encourages patient to continue breathing diaphragmatically	a. Patient instructed to continue performing procedure
		b. Patient informed of potential benefits

APE 7.2 Pursed Lip Breathing		
Performance	**Essential Tasks**	**Evaluation Criteria**
A. Demonstrate Procedure	1. Instructs patient to observe demonstration 2. Performs the following: • Inhales slowly through nose • Exhales slowly through pursed lips	a. Clear and accurate instructions provided a. Procedure demonstrated correctly
B. Coach Patient	1. Instructs patient to: • Inhale slowly through nose • Exhale slowly through pursed lips	a. Clear and accurate instructions provided
C. Complete Procedure	1. Repeats breathing instructions 2. Encourages patient to continue breathing through pursed lips	a. Previous step repeated until procedure mastered or patient tires a. Patient instructed to continue performing procedure b. Patient informed of potential benefits

APE 7.3 Cough Assist		
Performance	**Essential Tasks**	**Evaluation Criteria**
A. Demonstrate Procedure	1. Instructs patient to observe demonstration	a. Clear and accurate instructions provided
	2. Performs the following: • Places hands on abdomen beneath ribcage • Moves abdomen out while inhaling • Pushes hands up and in during cough	a. Procedure demonstrated correctly
B. Position Patient	1. Patient placed supine	a. Patient supine
C. Coach Patient	1. Places hands under ribcage on abdomen	a. Clear and accurate instruction provided
	2. Instructs patient to inhale deeply	b. Universal precautions followed
	3. Instructs patient to cough forcefully	
	4. Applies simultaneous upward thrust with cough effort	
	5. Assists with secretion removal	
D. Complete Procedure	1. Repeats instructions	a. Previous steps repeated until repeated until procedure mastered or patient tires
	2. Encourages patient to request cough assist as needed	a. Patient instructed to request procedure as needed

Module 8.0

Airway Care

A major responsibility of the respiratory care practitioner involves assessment and management of the patient's airway. This includes removal of secretions, maintenance of artificial airways and removal of artificial airways that are no longer needed. The purpose of this module is to ensure your proficiency in the performance of suctioning procedures, tracheostomy care, cuff pressure monitoring, pharyngeal airway insertion, and extubation.

Objectives

Upon completion of this module, you will be able to:

1. List the indications and hazards of suctioning.

2. List the indications and hazards of extubation.

3. Perform nasotracheal and endotracheal suctioning procedures without assistance.

4. Perform the procedures required for routine care of an artifical airway used in tracheostomy patients.

5. Perform extubation procedures without assistance.

6. Describe the indications for pharyngeal airway insertion.

7. Perform pharyngeal airway insertion without assistance.

8. Discuss the technique for monitoring and maintaining endotracheal cuff pressure.

9. Monitor and maintain the endotracheal cuff pressure for a patient who has been intubated.

Without an open and functioning airway, it is impossible to maintain life for more than a few minutes. Several procedures are performed clinically to remove or bypass obstructions which tend to reduce airway patency. These procedures include suctioning to remove copious secretions and the insertion of artificial airways into the respiratory tract. Oropharyngeal and nasopharyngeal airways are used to bypass or prevent upper airway obstruction in patients with no apparent respiratory distress. In other airway obstruction situations, particularly those requiring ventilatory assistance for the patient, an endotracheal or tracheostomy tube must be inserted into the airway.

The process of inserting an endotracheal tube, either orally or nasally, into the lower portion of the trachea is known as intubation. Except in hospitals where experienced respiratory therapists are allowed to intubate patients, this procedure is performed by a physician.

The insertion of an endotracheal tube almost always causes some epithelial damage to the airway. The results of this damage can vary from slight hoarseness to tracheal malacia and stenosis. The provision of proper airway care includes efforts to minimize tracheal damage caused by the intubation and movement of the tube once it is inserted. Because airway damage can also result from excessive pressure inside the cuff of the tube, it is important to maintain the cuff at as low a pressure as possible.

When a patient cannot be intubated, or when an artificial airway is required for more than a few days, a tracheostomy is performed. A tracheostomy involves the placement of an artifical airway in the trachea through a surgical incision made at the level of the second or third tracheal cartilage. A tracheostomy tube is inserted into the surgical opening and held in place by means of special tracheostomy ties. Respiratory care personnel are responsible for providing routine care following a tracheostomy.

Ancillary Procedure 8.1
Tracheal Suctioning

Tracheal suctioning is performed to remove accumulated secretions from the airway. When performing the procedure, a suction catheter is inserted into the trachea and a vacuum applied. An intermittent pressure of -80 to -120 mmHg (-60 to -80 mmHg for children) is applied for a period of 10 to 15 seconds while continuously monitoring the patient for adverse responses. Care must be taken to maintain sterile technique and to minimize mucosal damage when performing tracheal suctioning. Because tracheal suctioning necessitates exposure to body fluids, universal precautions are paramount during the procedure.

Indications

Tracheal suctioning is useful in patients who are incapable of mobilizing secretions of the lower respiratory tract. This includes patients with artificial airways, those unable to cough effectively due to a disease process such as myasthenia gravis or Guillain-Barré syndrome and those with decreased cough reflex due to such factors as coma or drug overdose.

Hazards and Complications

The potential hazards associated with airway suctioning include acute hypoxemia, cardiac arrhythmias, bradycardia, hypotension, atelectasis and infection. In order to minimize these adverse effects, the patient should always be hyperoxygenated before and after the suctioning process. In addition, if the need for further suctioning is evident, the entire process should be repeated rather than extending the time of each application.

Procedure for Suctioning

It is recommended that tracheal suctioning of a patient be performed according to the following procedure:

A. *Maintain Asepsis.* While performing the remainder of this procedure, you are expected to maintain aspetic conditions and follow universal precautions according to the procedure described in **SSE 1.2**. This includes the following:

1. Wash your hands:

    • Before obtaining equipment
    • Following performance of *H. Conclude Procedure*
    • Anytime during the procedure that contamination is suspected

2. Take universal precautions whenever the possiblity of exposure of body fluids exist by wearing:

    • Gloves
    • Mask
    • Eye protection

B. *Obtain Equipment.* Collect the following equipment and supplies:

• Suction Machine
• Connective tubing
• Sterile suction catheters
• Sterile gloves
• Sterile water
• Sterile container
• Stethoscope
• Eye protection
• Mask

C. *Assemble Equipment.* Prepare the equipment for use as follows:

1. Connect the tubing to the suction machine outlet.

2. Plug the suction machine into the vacuum wall outlet.

D. *Test Equipment.* Test the suctioning equipment as follows:

1. Turn on the vacuum control.

2. Fill the cup with water and insert the tip of the connective tubing into the water

3. If water does not enter the collection bottle:

   • Tighten all connections
   • Increase the vacuum (not more than -120 mmHg)

4. If water still does not enter the collection bottle:

   a. Label the suction equipment as "defective" and replace it.
   b. Reassemble and retest the new equipment.

E. *Confirm Patient.* Ensure that the procedure is performed with the correct patient as follows:

1. Match the information on the order with the following:

   • Room number
   • Name on the door or bed
   • Name on the wristband

2. Greet the patient by name (in a questioning manner if unknown).

3. Resolve any discrepancies in the patient identification information by conferring with the nursing staff.

F. *Inform Patient.* Interact with the patient as follows:

1. Introduce yourself by name and department (if not already acquainted).

2. Tell the patient what procedure is to be performed.

3. Explain the procedure by describing:

   • Why it is to be performed
   • How it will be performed
   • What the patient is expected to do
   • What you will be doing
   • How frequently it will be performed

Notes

G. *Implement Procedure.* Perform the following tasks:

1. Check the patient's pulse rate:

   - Before the procedure
   - During the procedure (if patient is connected to a heart monitor)
   - Following the procedure

2. If trachycardia or bradycardia occur, stop the procedure.

3. Adjust the vacuum between -80 and 120 mmHg (-60 and -80 mm Hg for children).

4. Hyperoxygenate the patient by:

   - Increasing the oxygen concentration
                        or
   - Instructing the patient to breathe deeply (or sighing the patient if receiving ventilatory assistance)

5. Put on gloves, mask, and eye protection according to the standard operating procedure.

6. Attach the sterile catheter tip to the connective tubing.

7. Without applying suction, insert the catheter into the mouth, nose or trachea to a point of restriction.

8. While removing the catheter, rotate and apply intermittent suction for no longer than 15 seconds.

H. *Conclude Procedure.* Complete the following tasks:

1. Clear the suction tubing with water and turn off the suction machine.

2. Aseptically dispose of the gloves, mask, eye protection, and catheter.

3. Auscultate the patient's chest according to the procedure described in **SSE 2.2**. Repeat suctioning if audible rales are present.

4. Place the patient in a comfortable position.

5. Assure that the call bell and bedside table are within the patient's reach.

6. Ask if the patient has any needs.

7. Answer any questions as effectively as possible.

I. ***Record Results.*** Document the therapy as follows:

1. Record the following data on the patient's chart:

   • Date
   • Time
   • Procedure
   • Color, amount and consistency of sputum
   • Abnormal patient characteristics
   • Therapy-related patient complaints

2. Sign the patient's chart (first initial and full last name).

J. ***Report Observations.*** Report the following information:

1. Report any significant adverse changes in the patient's condition to the nurse or physician whenever observed.

2. Following the procedure, inform the appropriate personnel of:

   • Patient requests
   • Patient complaints
   • Unexpressed patient needs

3. Following the procedure, report to the nurse or physician:

   • Any non-critical adverse reactions to the therapy
   • Other pertinent observations of the patient's condition

Ancillary Procedure 8.2
Tracheostomy Care

Tracheostomy is the surgical creation of an opening into the trachea of a patient. This opening in the neck requires routine care to minimize the risk of infection. Such care involves cleaning the opening (stoma) and changing the surgical dressing at least three times a day. Since a tracheostomy is ordinarily perfomed in the treatment of some serious patient condition, it is extremely important that infection of the stoma or other complications related to the creation of the artificial airway be avoided.

Indications

A change of the tracheal dressing is indicated by the presence of secretions on the dressing. Otherwise, the dressing should be changed every eight hours as a matter of routine. Any changes in the appearance of the stoma which suggest the possibility of infection should be reported to the nurse or physician.

Hazards and Precautions

When changing a tracheostomy dressing, care should be taken to avoid undue stress on the tracheal stoma and to prevent inadvertant expulsion of the tracheostomy tube. To minimize these potential problems, it is desirable to obtain assistance while changing the dressing. In case of airway obstruction or respiratory difficulty, it is also advisable to have a manual resuscitator with an oxygen source readily available at bedside. Although such problems seldom occur, suitable precautions should always be taken.

Procedure for Tracheostomy Care

It is recommended that the following procedure be followed when performing tracheostomy care for a patient:

A.   *Maintain Asepsis.* While performing the remainder of this procedure, you are expected to maintain aseptic conditions and follow universal precautions according to the procedure described in **SSE 1.2**. This includes the following:

1. Wash your hands:

   - Before obtaining equipment
   - Following performance of *F. **Conclude Procedure***
   - Anytime during the procedure that contamination is suspected

2. Take universal precautions whenever the possibility of exposure to body fluids exists by wearing:

   - Gloves
   - Mask
   - Eye Protection

B. ***Obtain Equipment.*** Collect the following equipment and supplies:

   - Sterile tracheostomy dressing
   - Cotton swabs
   - Tracheostomy tape
   - Hydrogen peroxide
   - Sterile container for hydrogen peroxide
   - Hemostat
   - Stethoscope
   - Resuscitation bag
   - Oxygen supply
   - Gloves, mask, and eye protection

C. ***Confirm Patient.*** Ensure that the procedure is performed with the correct patient as follows:

1. Match the information on the order with the following:

   - Room number
   - Name on the door or bed
   - Name on the wristband

2. Greet the patient by name (in a questioning manner if unknown).

3. Resolve any discrepancies in the patient identification information by conferring with the nursing staff.

D. ***Inform Patient.*** Interact with the patient as follows:

1. Introduce yourself by name and department (if not already acquainted).

2. Tell the patient what procedure is to be performed.

Notes

3. Explain the procedure by describing:

- Why it is to be performed
- How it will be performed
- What the patient is expected to do
- What you will be doing
- How frequently it will be performed

E. **Implement Procedure.** Perform the following tasks:

1. Wash your hands according to the procedure described in **SSE 1.1**.

2. Put on gloves, mask, and eye protection according to the standard operating procedure.

3. Position the patient's neck to facilitate access to the trachea.

4. Remove the tracheostomy ties and dressing while an assistant maintains tube placement.

5. Gently clean the tracheostomy stoma with hydrogen peroxide and cotton swabs while an assistant maintains tube placement. If a double lumen tracheostomy tube is employed, clean the inner cannula and rinse it with sterile water.

6. Aseptically remove the gloves and put on another pair of sterile gloves according to the standard operating procedure.

7. Place the sterile tracheostomy dressing around the tracheostomy tube and secure the tube with tracheostomy ties. (Tracheostomy ties should be tight enough to allow only two fingers between the neck and the tracheostomy tube. A square knot should be used to secure the tracheostomy ties.)

F. **Conclude Procedure.** Complete the following tasks:

1. Aseptically dispose of the gloves, mask, and eye protection.

2. Auscultate the patient's chest.

3. Place the patient in a comfortable position.

4. Assure that the call bell and bedside table are within the patient's reach.

5. Ask if the patient has any needs.

6. Answer any questions as effectively as possible

. G. Record Results. Document the therapy as follows:

    1. Record the following data on the patient's chart:

- Date
- Time
- Procedure
- Color, amount and consistency of sputum
- Abnormal patient characteristics
- Therapy-related patient complaints

    2. Sign the patient's chart (first initial and full last name).

H. *Report Observations.* Report the following information:

    1. Report any significant adverse changes in the patient's condition to the nurse or physician whenever observed.

    2. Following the procedure, inform the appropriate personnel of:

- Patient requests
- Patient complaints
- Unexpressed patient needs

    3. Following the procedure, report to the nurse or physician:

- Any non-critical adverse reactions to the therapy
- Other pertinent observations of the patient's condition

Ancillary Procedure 8.3
Endotracheal Extubation

The process of removing an endotracheal tube, known as extubation, is often performed by respiratory care personnel. During extubation, it is necessary to perform several preliminary procedures before actually removing the endotracheal tube. These procedures include suctioning the trachea and the oropharynx and completely deflating the endotraceal tube cuff. To assist with further removal of secretions, the endotracheal tube can be removed with a suction catheter inserted in the tube and with suction applied during removal. The patient is immediately administered oxygen, encouraged to breathe deeply and cough.

Indications

Extubation is performed when the indications which led to the insertion of an artificial airway are no longer present. If the airway was needed to bypass an upper airway obstruction, extubation is initiated when the patient shows signs that the obstruction has been reduced. These signs include a visible reduction in swelling or an improvement in sensorium. If intubation was performed for administration of mechanical ventilation, the artifical airway can be removed when the patient has no futher need for ventilatory support. This status is evidenced by adequate improvement in the patient's ventilatory status and blood gas values.

Hazards and Precautions

Since reinsertion of the endotracheal tube is sometimes necessary, extubation should only be performed by, or in the presence of, personnel qualified to perfom intubation. Equipment necessary for reintubation and a manual resuscitation bag must also be readily available. The patient should be closely evaluated for any signs of airway obstruction or respiratory distress. Monitoring of the patient is continued until it is certain that the artificial airway is no longer needed.

Procedure for Performing Endotracheal Extubation

It is recommended that the following procedure be used for endotracheal extubation:

A. ***Check Order.*** Verify the physician's order as follows:

    1. Compare the requisition with the physician's order to ensure that no discrepancies exist.

    2. Review the order to ensure that the following are prescribed:

        • Physician's order for extubation
        • Post-extubation oxygen delivery device
        • Gas flow rate or FIO_2

    3. If any part of the order is unfamiliar, question its accuracy.

B. ***Review Chart.*** Use the following procedure to review the patient's chart:

    1. On the patient's chart, identify all pertinent data in the following areas:

        • History and physical
        • Admitting diagnosis
        • Progress notes
        • Blood gas analysis

C. ***Maintain Asepsis.*** While performing the remainder of this procedure, you are expected to maintain aseptic conditions and follow universal precautions according to the procedure described in **SSE 1.2**.

    1. Wash your hands:

        • Before obtaining equipment
        • Following performance of ***K. Conclude Procedure***
        • Anytime during the procedure that contamination is suspected

    2. Taking universal precautions whenever the possibility of exposure to body fluids exists by wearing:

        • Gloves
        • Mask
        • Eye Protection

D. *Obtain Equipment.* Collect the following equipment and supplies:

- Stethoscope
- Scissors
- Syringe
- Suctioning equipment
- Oxygen delivery equipment
- Oxygen analyzer
- Gloves, mask, and eye protection

E. *Assemble Equipment.* Using the standard operating procedures, assemble:

- Suctioning equipment (**APE 8.1**)
- Oxygen delivery equipment (**CPE 9.1** or **CPE 10.1**)

F. *Test Equipment.* Using the standard operating procedures, test:

- Suctioning equipment (**APE 8.1**)
- Oxygen delivery equipment (**CPE 9.1** or **CPE 10.1**)

G. *Confirm Patient.* Ensure that the procedure is performed with the correct patient as follows:

1. Match the information on the order with the following:

   - Room number
   - Name on the door or bed
   - Name on the wristband

2. Greet the patient by name (in a questioning manner if unknown).

3. Resolve any discrepancies in the patient identification information by conferring with the nursing staff.

H. *Inform Patient.* Interact with the patient as follows:

1. Introduce yourself by name and department (if not already acquainted).

2. Tell the patient what procedure is to be performed.

3. Explain the procedure by describing:

   - Why it is to be performed
   - How it will be performed
   - What the patient is expected to do
   - What you will be doing
   - How frequently it will be performed

I. Implement Procedure. Perform the following tasks:

    1. Using the standard operating procedure (**APE 8.1**), suction the:

- Trachea
- Oropharynx

    2. While an assistant removes the endotracheal tube ties and maintains placement of the tube, thoroughly deflate the endotracheal tube cuff.

    3. Extubate the patient by:

- Inserting a sterile catheter into the trachea
- Applying suction on removal
- Removing the catheter and endotracheal tube simultaneously

            or

- Ask the patient to inhale and quickly but gently remove the tube

    4. Encourage the patient to breathe deeply and cough:

- Immediately following removal of the tube
- Frequently while excessive secretions are present

    5. Administer oxygen according to the standard operating procedure (**CPE .1** or **CPE 10.1**)

J. Monitor Patient. Determine the patient's response to therapy as follows:

    1. Determine pulse rate. (Count for a minimum of one minute.)

    2. Determine the respiratory rate. (Count for a minimum of one minute.)

    3. Observe respiration to identify any abnormalities in the breathing pattern.

    4. Ausculate the patient's chest according to the procedure described in **SSE 2.2**.

    5. Note any abnormalities in the patient's appearance or behavior.

K. *Conclude Procedure.* Complete the following tasks:

1. Place the patient in a comfortable position.

2. Assure that the call bell and bedside table are within the patient's reach.

3. Ask if the patient has any needs.

4. Answer any questions as effectively as possible.

L. *Record Results.* Document the therapy as follows:

1. Record the following data on the patient's chart:

   • Date
   • Time
   • Procedure
   • Color, amount and consistency of sputum
   • Abnormal patient characteristics
   • Therapy-related patient complaints

2. Sign the patient's chart (first initial and full last name).

M. *Report Observations.* Report the following information.

1. Report any significant adverse changes in the patient's condition to the nurse or physician whenever observed.

2. Following the procedure, inform the appropriate personnel of:

   • Patient requests
   • Patient complaints
   • Unexpressed patient needs

3. Following the procedure, report to the nurse or physician:

   • Any non-critical adverse reactions to the therapy
   • Other pertinent observations of the patient's condition

Ancillary Procedure 8.4
Endotracheal Tube Cuff
Pressure Maintenance

The artificial airway used with most patients is an endotracheal tube with a pressurized cuff that is inflated to seal the airway. It is important that the pressure in the cuff be high enough to prevent the leaking of gas around the tube while respiration is maintained by mechanical ventilation. It is equally important, however, that the cuff pressure not be so high as to restrict circulation to the tracheal tissue around the cuff. Cuff pressures should be high enough to seal the airway but should never be maintained at a pressure higher than 20 cm H_2O.

Indications

When caring for a patient with a cuffed endotracheal tube, the pressure within the cuff should be monitored at least every eight hours. In addition, the cuff pressure should be checked at any time that a leak is suspected. The cuff should remain fully inflated at all times unless otherwise ordered by the physician. A properly inflated cuff is necessary to prevent the aspiration of oral secretions into the lungs as well as to prevent the leakage of air around the tube.

Potential Hazards

The primary risks associated with the maintenance of endotracheal tube cuff pressure have already been mentioned. If the cuff pressure is too low, a leak will occur around the endotracheal tube, and the patient may receive inadequate ventilation. If the pressure is too high, the cuff will interfere with circulation in the blood vessels of the trachea. Total occlusion of the blood vessels will. Anytime that it is not possible to seal the trachea at a pressure below 20 cm H_2O, the nurse or physician should be notified immediately.

Procedure for Monitoring Cuff Pressure

It is recommended that cuff pressure monitoring be performed according to the following procedure:

A. **Check Order.** Verify the physician's order as follows:

1. Compare the requisition with the physician's order to ensure that no discrepancies exist.

2. If any part of the order is unfamiliar, question its accuracy.

B. **Maintain Asepsis.** While performing the remainder of this procedure, you are expected to maintain aseptic conditions according to the procedures described in **SSE 1.2**. This includes the use of universal precautions and handwashing. Gloves must be worn during the actual procedure. Hands should be washed:

- Before obtaining equipment
- Following performance of step **G. Conclude Procedure**
- Anytime during the procedure that contamination is suspected.

C. **Obtain Equipment.** Collect the following equipment and supplies:

- Gloves
- Cuff Pressure Manometer
- 12 to 20 cc syringe
- Three-way stopcock
- Stethoscope

D. **Confirm Patient.** Ensure that the procedure is performed on the correct patient as follows:

1. Match the information on the order with the following:

- Room number
- Name on the door or bed
- Name on the wristband

2. Greet the patient by name (in a questioning manner if unknown).

3. Resolve any discrepancies in the patient identification information by conferring with the nursing staff.

E. ***Inform Patient.*** Interact with the patient as follows:

1. Introduce yourself by name and department (if not already acquainted).

2. Tell the patient what procedure is to be performed.

3. Explain the procedure by describing:

    - Why it is to be performed?
    - How it will be performed?
    - What the patient is expected to do?
    - What you will be doing?
    - How frequently it will be performed?

F. ***Implement Procedure.*** Perform the following tasks:

1. Attach the syringe (with plunger withdrawn 5-10 ml) to the pressure manometer via the three-way stopcock.

2. Close the stopcock to room air and allow it to remain open between the syringe and manometer.

3. Adjust the plunger of the syringe until the manometer reads 20 cm H_2O.

4. Attach the third outlet of the stopcock to the pilot line of the endotracheal tube.

5. Open the stopcock to allow communication between all three ports.

6. Auscultate the neck area over the trachea to identify any airleak.

7. Using the syringe, adjust the pressure within the system to the lowest possible level at which no leaks are heard.

8. Close the stopcock to the pilot line.

9. Remove the stopcock from the pilot line.

G. ***Conclude Procedure.*** Complete the following tasks:

1. Place the patient in a comfortable position.

2. Assure that the call bell and bedside table are within the patient's reach.

3. Ask if the patient has any needs.

4. Answer any questions as effectively as possible.

H.   ***Record Results.*** Record the following data on the patient chart as required:

- Patient name
- Room number
- Cuff Pressure
- Any adverse patient reactions

I.   ***Report Observations.*** Report the following information:

1. Report any significant adverse changes in the patient's condition to the nurse or physician.

2. Following the procedure, inform the appropriate personnel of:

   - Patient requests
   - Patient complaints
   - Unexpressed patient needs

3. Following the procedure, report to the nurse or physician:

   - Any non-critical adverse reactions to the therapy
   - Other pertinent observations of the patient's condition

Ancillary Procedure 8.5
Pharyngeal Airway Insertion

The most common cause of airway obstruction is the closing of the tracheal opening within the pharynx by the tongue or other soft tissue. When muscle tone is lost, the tongue has a tendency to fall back into the throat and occlude the airway. The tonsils, adenoids, and other soft tissues can swell and cause a narrowing of the tracheal opening. For this reason, pharyngeal airways are used to bypass soft tissue obstruction of the opening.

Pharyngeal airways can be divided into two categories: oropharyngeal airways and nasopharyngeal airways (nasal trumpets). The oral airway is designed to lift the tongue and physically hold it out of the opening of the trachea. The nasal trumpet is inserted through the nose, thus bypassing the tongue and providing a clear pathway for air to travel into the trachea.

Indications

Pharyngeal airways are indicated whenever there is evidence of upper airway obstruction or when the patient is observed to have a loss of muscle tone significant enough to lead to airway obstruction. Such loss is most likely to occur in situations where the patient is in an unconscious or semi-conscious state. In addition, nasal airways are indicated for the patient who requires frequent nasotracheal suctioning to prevent damage to the tracheal mucosa.

Hazards and Precautions

Oral airways are poorly tolerated by the fully conscious patient and will usually cause the patient to gag and spit the airway out. Fortunately, fully conscious patients generally have enough muscle tone that oral airways are not indicated.

An oral airway that is too large or too small can worsen the airway obstruction by further blocking the opening. For this reason, the airway must be properly sized and must only be used when it is indicated for an unconscious or semi-conscious patient. To assess the correct size for an oral airway, the length of the airway should match the distance between the tip of the chin and the top of the mandible, just beneath the ear.

Nasal airway insertion can be traumatic to the nasal mucosa if the airway is too large or not sufficiently lubricated. The correct size of airway can again be measured by looking at the distance between the chin and the mandible. However, the diameter of the airway should be small enough to fit easily within the diameter of the nostril. When inserting the airway, a water soluble lubricant should be used.

Procedure for Pharyngeal Airway Insertion

It is recommended that pharyngeal airway insertion be performed according to the following procedure:

A. *Check Order.* Verify the physician's order as follows:

  1. Compare the requisition with the physician's order to ensure that no discrepancies exist.

  2. If any part of the order is unfamiliar, question its accuracy.

B. *Maintain Asepsis.* While performing the remainder of this procedure, you are expected to maintain aseptic conditions according to the procedures described in **SSE 1.2**. This includes the use of universal precautions and handwashing. Gloves must be worn during the actual procedure. Hands should be washed:

  • Before obtaining equipment
  • Following performance of step **G. Conclude Procedure**
  • Anytime during the procedure that contamination is suspected.

C. *Obtain Equipment.* Collect the following equipment and supplies:

  • Gloves
  • Various sizes of oral or nasal airways (as applicable)
  • Water soluble lubricant

D. *Confirm Patient.* Ensure that the procedure is performed on the correct patient as follows:

  1. Match the information on the order with the following:

    • Room number
    • Name on the door or bed
    • Name on the wristband

  2. Greet the patient by name (in a questioning manner if unknown).

3. Resolve any discrepancies in the patient identification information by conferring with the nursing staff.

E. ***Inform Patient.*** If the patient is conscious, interact with him or her as follows:

1. Introduce yourself by name and department (if not already acquainted).

2. Tell the patient what procedure is to be performed.

3. Explain the procedure by describing:

    *   Why it is to be performed
    *   How it will be performed
    *   What the patient is expected to do
    *   What you will be doing
    *   How frequently it will be performed

F. ***Implement Procedure.*** Perform the following tasks:

1. Select the proper type and size of pharyngeal airway.

2. If an oral airway is to be used:

    a. Insert the airway into the mouth with the tip facing toward the roof of the mouth.

    b. Gently advance the airway into the mouth until the tip lies at the roof of the mouth.

    c. Rotate the airway until the tip is facing the tongue. Simultaneously, advance the airway completely into the mouth until the bite block is in front of the teeth.

    d. Secure the airway to the skin with tape as necessary to prevent dislodgement.

3. If a nasal airway is to be used:

    a. Generously lubricate the airway with water soluble jelly.

    b. Following the curvature of the nasal passage, gently advance the airway into one of the nostrils until the outer flange rests against the nostril opening.

c. If resistance is met, do not use excessive force. Instead, gently work the airway into the passage or reattempt insertion through the other nostril.

d. Attach a square of adhesive tape to the flange of the tube to prevent further slippage into the airway.

e. The airway may be left in place if frequent suctioning is required, but it must be removed and inserted in the other nostril every eight hours.

G. *Conclude Procedure.* Complete the following tasks:

1. Place the patient in a comfortable position.

2. Assure that the call bell and bedside table are within the patient's reach.

3. Ask if the patient has any needs.

4. Answer any questions as effectively as possible.

H. *Record Results.* Record the following data on the patient's chart as required:

• Patient name
• Room number
• Size airway used
• Any adverse patient reactions

I. *Report Observations.* Report the following information:

1. Report any significant adverse changes in the patient's condition to the nurse or physician.

2. Following the procedure, inform the appropriate personnel of:

• Patient requests
• Patient complaints
• Unexpressed patient needs

3. Following the procedure, report to the nurse or physician:

• Any non-critical adverse reactions to the therapy
• Other pertinent observations of the patient's condition

Evaluation of Airway Care Procedures

The following definitions are provided for use whenever the respective Airway Care Procedures are evaluated. In order for performance of the procedures to be considered acceptable, all Essential Tasks are to be performed according to the accompanying Evaluation Criteria. Any deviation from the following task sequence or criteria must be approved by the evaluator.

APE 8.1 Tracheal Suctioning		
Performance	**Essential Tasks**	**Evaluation Criteria**
A. Maintain Asepsis	See SSE 1.2	See SSE 1.2
B. Obtain Equipment	1. Obtains the following equipment and supplies: • Suction machine • Connective tubing • Sterile suction catheter • Sterile gloves • Sterile water • Sterile container • Stethoscope • Eye Protection • Mask	a. Correct equipment obtained
C. Assemble Equipment	1. Prepares equipment as follows: • Connects tubing to suction machine • Connects suction machine to vacuum source	a. Assembled according to **SOP**
D. Test Equipment	1. Tests for: • Leaks in system • Adequate suction	a. Tested according to b. Leaks remedied c. Defective equipment replaced
E. Confirm Patient	See SSE 3.3	See SSE 1.2
F. Inform Patient	See SSE 4.1	See SSE 4.1

APE 8.1
Tracheal Suctioning (continued)

Performance	Essential Tasks	Evaluation Criteria
G. Implement Procedure	1. Checks pulse rate: • Before procedure • During procedure (if patient connected to monitor) • Following procedure	a. Counted for at least one (1) minute b. Procedure stopped if tachycardia or bradycardia occur
	2. Adjusts vacuum	a. -80 to -120 mmHg (adults), or b. -60 to -80 mmHg (children)
	3. Hyperoxygenates patient	a. Oxygen increased b. Efforts made to get patient to breathe deeply by: • Instructing (if unassisted), or • Activating sighing control (if assisted)
	4. Puts on gloves, mask, and eye protection	a. According to **SOP** b. Sterility maintained
	5. Attaches catheter	a. Connected to tubing b. Sterility maintained
	6. Inserts catheter into: • Mouth, • Nose, or • Trachea	a. No suction applied b. Inserted to point of restriction
	7. Applies suction	a. Applied intermittently b. Time limit not exceeded c. Catheter removed d. Catheter rotate during removal
H. Conclude Procedure	1. Maintains Equipment	a. Protective attire and catheter aseptically disposed b. Suction tubing cleared c. Suction turned off
	2. Auscultates chest	a. Performed according to **SSE 2.2** b. Procedure repeated if rales audible
	3. Replaces call bell and bedside table	a. Placed within patient's reach
	4. Tends to patient needs	a. Comfortable position assured b. Patient asked regarding other needs

APE 8.1 Tracheal Suctioning (continued)		
Performance	**Essential Tasks**	**Evaluation Criteria**
H. Conclude Procedure (continued)		c. Patient questions answered effectively
I. Record Results	See SSE 3.4	See SSE 3.4
J. Report Observations	See SSE 4.3	See SSE 4.3

APE 8.2
Tracheostomy Care

Performance	Essential Tasks	Evaluation Criteria
A. Maintain Asepsis	See **SSE 1.2**	See **SSE 1.2**
B. Obtain Equipment	1. Obtains the following equipment and supplies: • Sterile tracheostomy dressing • Cotton swabs • Tracheostomy tape • Hydrogen peroxide • Hemostat • Stethoscope • Resuscitation bag • Oxygen supply	a. Correct equipment obtained
C. Confirm Patient	See **SSE 3.3**	See **SSE 1.2**
D. Inform Patient	See **SSE 4.1**	See **SSE 4.1**
E. Implement Procedure	1. Wash hands	a. Perform according to **SSE 1.1**
	2. Put on gloves, mask, and eye protection	a. According to **SOP** b. Sterility maintained
	3. Positions patient's neck	a. Trachea easily accessible
	4. Removes tracheostomy ties and dressing	a. Tube placement maintained
	5. Cleans tracheostomy stoma	a. Hydrogen peroxide used b. Cleaned thoroughly c. Tube placement maintained d. If double lumen tube, inner cannula cleaned and rinsed
	6. Changes gloves	a. According to **SOP** b. Sterility maintained
	7. Replaces dressing	a. Performed according to **SSE 1.2** b. Tube secured with tape c. Suitable knot used

APE 8.2 Tracheostomy Care (continued)		
Performance	**Essential Tasks**	**Evaluation Criteria**
E. Implement Procedure (continued)		d. Tape adjusted to correct tightness (two fingers between neck and tube)
F. Conclude Procedure	1. Disposes of gloves	a. Performed according to **SSE 1.2**
	2. Auscultates chest	a. Performed according to **SSE 2.2**
	3. Replaces call bell and bedside table	a. Placed within patient's reach
	4. Tends to patient needs	a. Comfortable position assured b. Patient asked regarding other needs c. Patient questions answered effectively
G. Record Results	See **SSE 3.4**	See **SSE 3.4**
H. Report Observations	See **SSE 4.3**	See **SSE 4.3**

APE 8.3
Endotracheal Extubation

Performance	Essential Tasks	Evaluation Criteria
A. Check Order	See SSE 3.1	See SSE 3.1
B. Review Chart	See SSE 3.2	See SSE 3.2
C. Maintain Asepsis	See SSE 1.2	See SSE 1.2
D. Obtain Equipment	1. Obtains the following equipment and supplies: • Stethoscope • Scissors • Syringe • Suctioning equipment • Oxygen delivery equipment • Oxygen analyzer	a. Correct equipment obtained
E. Assemble Equipment	1. Assembles suctioning equipment 2. Assembles oxygen delivery equipment	a. Performed according to APE 8.1 a. Performed according to CPE 9.1 or CPE 10.1
F. Test Equipment	1. Tests suctioning equipment 2. Tests oxygen delivery equipment equipment	a. Performed according to APE 8.1 a. Performed according to CPE9.1 or CPE 10.1
G. Confirm Patient	See SSE 3.3	See SSE 3.3
H. Inform Patient	See SSE 4.1	See SSE 4.1
I. Implement Procedure	1. Suctions: • Trachea • Oropharynx	a. Performed according to APE 8.1 to APE 8.1

APE 8.3
Endotracheal Extubation (continued)

Performance	Essential Tasks	Evaluation Criteria
I. Implement Procedure (continued)	2. Deflates endotracheal tube cuff	a. Tape removed (by assistant) b. Tube placement maintained (by assistant) b. Tube placement maintained (by assistant) c. Adequately deflated for removal
	3. Removes endotracheal tube	a. Sterile catheter inserted b. Catheter and tube removed simultaneously c. Suction applied on removal
	4. Patient encouraged to: • Breathe deeply • Cough	a. Instructions clear and complete b. Instructions repeated when needed
	5. Oxygen administered	a. Performed according to **CPE 9.1**
J. Monitor Patient	1. Determines: • Pulse rate • Respiratory rate	a. Counted for at least one (1) minute
	2. Observes: • Respiratory pattern • Patient appearance	a. Any abnormalties identified
	3. Auscultates chest	a. Performed according to **SSE 2.2**
K. Conclude Procedure	1. Replaces call bell and bedside table	a. Placed within patient's reach
	2. Tends to patient needs	a. Comfortable position assured b. Patient asked regarding other needs c. Patient questions answered effectively
L. Record Results	See **SSE 4.3**	See **SSE 4.3**
M. Report Observations	See **SSE 3.4**	See **SSE 3.4**

APE 8.4
Endotracheal Tube Cuff Pressure Maintenance

Performance	Essential Tasks	Evaluation Criteria
A. Check Order	See SSE 3.1	See SSE 3.1
B. Maintain Aspesis	See SSE 1.2	See SSE 1.2
C. Obtain Equipment	1. Obtains the following equipment: • Gloves • Pressure manometer • 12 - 20 cc syringe • 3-way stopcock • Stethoscope	a. Correct equipment obtained
D. Confirm Patient	See SSE 3.3	See SSE 3.3
E. Inform Patient	See SSE 4.1	See SSE 4.1
F. Implement Procedure	1. Attaches syringe to stopcock and manometer via stopcock	a. Syringe properly connected to manometer
	2. Adjusts system pressure to 20 cm H_2O	a. stopcock closed b. pressure in system at 20 cm H_2O
	3. Attaches third port to pilot line	a. Pilot line properly attached
	4. Opens pressurized system to pilot line	a. Pilot line opened to system without leakage
	5. Auscultates neck area for leak	a. Neck auscultated b. Any leak detected
	6. Adjusts to minimal leak	a. Pressure adjusted to minimum leak
	7. Closes stopcock to pilot line	a. Stopcock closed
	8. Removes stopcock from pilot line	a. Stopcock removed

APE 8.4		
Endotracheal Tube Cuff Pressure Maintenance (continued)		
Performance	**Essential Tasks**	**Evaluation Criteria**
G. Conclude Procedure	1. Replaces call bell and bedside 2. Tends to patient needs	a. Placed within patient's reach a. Comfortable position assured b. Patient asked regarding needs c. Patient questions answered effectively
H. Record Results	See **SSE 3.4**	See **SSE 3.4**
I. Report Observations	See **SSE 4.3**	See **SSE 4.3**

APE 8.5		
Pharyngeal Airway Insertion		
Performance	**Essential Tasks**	**Evaluation Criteria**
A. Check Order Order	See SSE 3.1	See SSE 3.1
B. Maintain Asepsis	See SSE 1.2	See SSE 1.2
C. Obtain Equipment	1. Obtains the following equipment • Gloves • Various sized pharyngeal airways • Water soluble lubricant	a. Correct equipment obtained
D. Confirm Patient	See SSE 3.3	See SSE 3.3
E. Inform Patient	See SSE 4.1	See SSE 4.1
F. Implement Procedure	1. Selects proper size airway	a. Proper size selected
	2. Inserts oral airway when indicated	a. Inserted in mouth with top facing up b. Advance until tip is at roof of mouth c. Tip rotated towards tongue and advanced to bite block d. Airway properly secured
	3. Inserts nasal airway when indicated	a. Generously lubricate b. Airway advanced gently c. Advance through nare until flange is at nostril d. If resistance met, gentle pressure used or insertion attemped with opposite nare e. Airway secured properly f. Site changed every eight hours and as needed

APE 8.5 Pharyngeal Airway Insetion (continued)		
Performance	**Essential Tasks**	**Evaluation Criteria**
G. Conclude Procedure	1. Replaces call bell and bedside table	a. Placed within patient's reach
	2. Tends to patient needs	a. Comfortable position assured b. Patient asked regarding needs c. Patient's questions answered effectively
H. Record Results	See **SSE 3.4**	See **SSE 3.4**
I. Report Observations	See **SSE 4.3**	See **SSE 4.3**

Section Three
Clinical Procedures

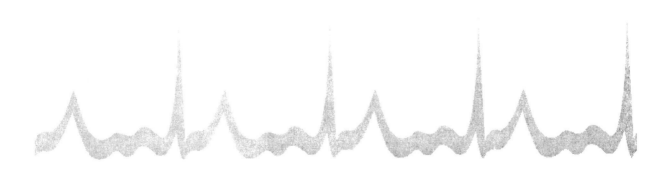

Module 9.0

Oxygen Therapy

Oxygen is an odorless, tasteless gas that is essential to life. It makes up approximately 21% of the air that we breathe. Higher concentrations of oxygen may have a therapeutic effect on certain patient conditions. Whenever the gas exchange process in the body is impaired and the levels of oxygen in the bloodstream are low, oxygen therapy should be initiated to bring the oxygen level back to normal. Oxygen can be delivered to the body in a variety of ways. This module deals specifically with the procedures used to administer oxygen therapy.

Objectives

Upon completion of this module, you will be able to:

1. List and explain the conditions that indicate the use of oxygen therapy.

2. List and describe the potential hazards associated with oxygen therapy.

3. Compare the characteristics of different oxygen delivery devices and describe the major advantages and disadvantages of each.

4. Assemble and test all equipment necessary for the delivery of supplemental oxygen.

5. Administer oxygen therapy according to the procedure prescribed for a patient.

Clinical Procedure 9.1
Oxygen Therapy

Oxygen therapy refers to the administration of oxygen-enriched air to a patient. The immediate effect of increasing a patient's fraction of inspired oxygen (FIO_2) is an increase in alveolar oxygen tension. For this reason, oxygen therapy is an effective treatment for hypoxemia that results from decreased alveolar oxygen tension. Because hypoxemia tends to cause increased heart rate and respiratory rate, this treatment may further benefit a patient by reducing myocardial work and work of breathing.

Oxygen can be administered in concentrations up to 100%. The specific concentration prescribed depends on the patient's condition and the therapeutic goal. These factors are determined by measurement of arterial blood gases and evaluation of cardiopulmonary status. Similar assessments are made routinely during oxygen administration to determine the adequacy and effectiveness of therapy.

The administration of a dry gas such as oxygen can create a humidity deficit for the patient unless preventive measures are taken. For this reason, a humidifier is used to add water vapor to the gas delivered to the patient, especially when the flow rate is 3 lm or more.

Indications

Respiratory care personnel should be thoroughly familiar with the conditions that indicate the need for supplemental oxygen. Some of the commonly occurring causes of hypoxemia that are treated by oxygen therapy are the following:

1. Pulmonary insufficiency due to conditions such as chronic obstructive pulmonary disease, asthma, or pneumonia.

2. Reduced cardiovascular efficiency due to conditions such as myocardial infarction, cardiac arrest, or shock.

3. Reduced efficiency of skeletal muscles that aid in respiration due to conditions such as drug overdose, Guillain-Barré syndrome, or myasthenia gravis.

4. Noxious gas poisoning resulting from inhalation of gases such as smoke, carbon monoxide, or gasoline fumes.

Some of the clinical signs associated with hypoxemia are:

- Increased respiratory rate
- Increased heart rate
- Disorientation
- Diaphoresis
- Cyanosis

Hazards and Precautions

Oxygen administered in high concentrations can have harmful as well as beneficial effects. This is particularly true for patients receiving oxygen for extended periods of time. The potential hazards of oxygen therapy include the following:

1. Oxygen-induced hypoventilation, especially in patients with chronic obstructive pulmonary disease.

2. Absorption atelectasis caused by an increased partial pressure of oxygen accompanied by a decreased partial pressure of nitrogen.

3. Oxygen toxicity, particularly of lung tissue, caused by inspiring a high concentration of oxygen over an extended period of time.

4. Neonatal retrolental fibroplasia caused by high partial pressures of oxygen in arterial blood.

Because of the potential hazards of oxygen therapy, the concentration and the duration of delivery of oxygen should be closely monitored. Care should be taken to limit delivery to the level needed to produce the desired therapeutic results. Keep in mind, however, that none of the hazards of oxygen therapy pose as great an immediate threat to the patient as the effects of dangerous levels of hypoxemia.

There is one additional potential hazard associated with the delivery of oxygen. Whenever the concentration of oxygen is increased, the risk of fire is similarly increased. Every precaution should be taken to restrict smoking and to avoid the presence of anything that could create a spark or otherwise ignite combustible materials in an oxygen-enriched environment.

Oxygen Delivery Equipment

There are two types of oxygen delivery systems, high-flow and low-flow. A high-flow system provides the entire gas flow inspired by a patient, while a low-flow system does not. In order to provide sufficient gas to meet the inspiratory requirements, a low-flow system utilizes room air to supplement the gas supplied by the system. As a result, the FIO_2 delivered at a given rate with a low-flow system varies with the patient's tidal volume and respiratory rate and pattern. With a high-flow system, the gas is delivered at a controlled FIO_2 and is not affected by changes in the patient's respiratory pattern.

There are several different devices available for delivering supplemental oxygen with each system. Selection of the proper system and device depends on the needs and condition of the patient. *Table 9-1* compares the characteristics of the most common oxygen delivery devices.

Table 9-1
Oxygen Delivery Devices

A low-flow system is ordinarily used for oxygen delivery if it is considered adequate for the patient's needs. It is less expensive and more convenient to operate that a high-flow system.

Delivery System	Delivery Device	Delivers Total FIO_2	Delivers Relatively Constant FIO_2	Approximate Oxygen Concentration Delivered	Gas Flow	Relative Patient Comfort	Other Considerations
Low Flow	Nasal Cannula	No	No	25-50%	1-6 LPM	High	Cannot be used unless nasal passages are patent
	Nasal Catheter	No	No	25-50%	1-6 LPM	Moderate	Must be changed at lease every eight hours
	Simple Mask	No	No	35-50%	5-8 LPM	Moderate	
	Partial Rebreathing Mask	No	No	55-70%	6-10 LPM	Moderate	Reservoir bag should remain at least one-third full at all times in order to deliver desired FIO_2
	Non-rebreathing Mask	No	No	90-100%	6-10 LPM	Moderate	Reservoir bag should remain at least one-third full at all times in order to deliver desired FIO_2
High Flow	Venturi Mask	Yes	Yes	25-50%	Varies with manufacturer	Moderate	Device of choice for patients with COPD and hypo-ventilation syndrome
	Nebulizer	Yes	Yes	25-100%	10-12 LPM	Low	Provides controlled temperature and humidity of inspired gas

Furthermore, the delivery devices which are most commonly used with a low-flow system are more comfortable for the patient. The factors which determine the adequacy of a low-flow system are the patient's tidal volume, respiratory rate and breathing pattern. The breathing pattern must be regular and consistent, and the respiratory rate and tidal volume must be within acceptable limits. (Acceptable limits vary among patients. For the adult patient, a tidal volume of at least 300 ml and a respiratory rate of no more than 25 per minute is acceptable.)

Once it has been decided that a low-flow system will provide adequate ventilation, the next factor to consider is the selection of a delivery device. This decision is influenced primarily by the patient. When the patient's supplementary oxygen requirement is low, a nasal cannula, nasal catheter or simple mask may be used. Since a nasal cannula is simpler to apply and more comfortable for the patient, it is the device of choice unless the nasal passages are closed or it is likely to be displaced by the patient. For moderate oxygen concentrations, a simple mask is used as the delivery device. To deliver high concentrations of oxygen, it is necessary to use a nonrebreathing or a partial-rebreathing mask.

In situation where a consistent and predictable level of oxygen is required, it is necessary to employ a high-flow delivery system. The most commonly used device for delivering low concentrations of inspired oxygen with a high-flow system is the venturi mask. If the device is required for several days or if an aerosol is required along with oxygen, a nebulizer utilizing the Bernoulli principle may be used. (The nebulizer is mentioned at this time for the sake of completeness. Since it is more frequently used for aerosol therapy, however, it is addressed in greater detail in the next module.)

The device used for administering oxygen therapy is usually prescribed by the physician. We have provided a simple description of the basic guidelines followed in the selection of such a device. In general, the selection decision is most influenced by the concentration of oxygen required by the patient. It is also important, however, to give consideration to patient comfort. A mask capable of delivering the desired oxygen concentration is useless if the patient refuses to wear it because it is too hot or because it causes a feeling of suffocation. If this occurs, the physician should be contacted in order that an alternative device can be considered.

When administering oxygen therapy, the patient should be routinely monitored in order to detect changes in status which may have implications for the therapy. In addition, the physician may order arterial blood gas analysis in order to detect changes in status which may have implications for the therapy. In addition, the physician may order arterial blood gas analysis in order to determine the adequacy of oxygenation. Any changes in the patient's blood gas results, vital signs, respiratory pattern or appearance should be noted and brought to the attention of the physician. As a result of the information collected through patient monitoring, changes in the concentration of oxygen or the delivery device may be ordered.

Procedure for Oxygen Therapy

It is recommended that the following procedure be used for administering prescribed oxygen to a patient:

A. ***Check Order.*** Verify the physician's order as follows:

   1. Compare the requisition with the physician's order to ensure that no discrepancies exist.

   2. Review the order to ensure that the following are prescribed:

      • Oxygen delivery device
      • Gas flow rate or FIO_2
      • Frequency of therapy

   3. If any part of the order is unfamiliar, question its accuracy.

B. ***Review Chart.*** Use the following procedure to review the patient's chart:

   1. On the patient's chart, identify all pertinent data in the following areas:

      • History and physical
      • Admitting diagnosis
      • Progress notes
      • Blood-gas analysis

   2. Based on the patient data, identify the following:

      • Conditions that indicate the need for oxygen therapy
      • Potential hazards of oxygen therapy for the patient
      • Major advantages and disadvantages of the prescribed delivery device

C. ***Maintain Asepsis.*** While performing the remainder of this procedure, you are expected to maintain aseptic conditions and follow universal precautions according to the procedure described in **SSE 1.2**. This includes washing your hands:

   • Before obtaining equipment
   • Following performance of step ***K. Conclude Procedure***
   • Anytime during the procedure that contamination is suspected

D. *Obtain Equipment.* Collect the following equipment and supplies:

- Oxygen flowmeter
- Humidifier (as applicable)
- Sterile water
- Oxygen-supply tubing
- Prescribed delivery device
- "No Smoking" signs

E. *Assemble Equipment.* Prepare the equipment for use as follows:

1. Fill the humidifier to the mark with water.

2. Attach the oxygen supply tubing to the humidifier outlet.

3. Attach the other end of the supply tubing to the oxygen delivery device.

4. Connect the oxygen flowmeter to the gas inlet of the humidifier.

F. *Test Equipment.* Test the oxygen-delivery equipment as follows:

1. Connect the flowmeter to the outlet of the oxygen supply.

2. Turn on the flowmeter.

3. Stop the flow of gas by pinching the oxygen-supply tubing.

4. If the high-pressure alarm does not sound, check the system for leaks.

5. Stop any leaks by ensuring proper fit of all connections.

6. If the alarm is still not activated:

   a. Label the humidifier as *defective* and replace it.
   b. Reassemble and retest the new equipment.

G. *Confirm Patient.* Ensure that the procedure is performed with the correct patient as follows:

1. Match the information on the order with the following:

   - Room number
   - Name on the door or bed
   - Name on the wristband

2. Greet the patient by name (in a questioning manner if unknown).

3. Resolve any discrepancies in the patient identification information by conferring with the nursing staff.

H. *Inform Patient.* Interact with the patient as follows:

1. Introduce yourself by name and department (if not already acquainted).

2. Tell the patient what procedure is to be performed.

3. Explain the procedure by describing:

   • Why it is to be performed
   • How it will be performed
   • What the patient is expected to do
   • What you will be doing
   • How frequently it will be performed

4. Explain the fire hazards associated with the use of oxygen and caution against smoking.

I. *Implement Procedure.* Perform the following tasks:

1. Post "No Smoking" signs above the patient's bed and on the door.

2. Administer oxygen therapy as follows:

   a. Adjust the flowmeter to the prescribed gas-flow rate.
   b. Adjust the oxygen-delivery device to the patient.
   c. Ensure that the delivery device fits comfortably.
   d. If a mask with a reservoir bag is used, be certain that the bag remains at least one-third full at all times.

J. *Monitor Patient.* Determine the patient's response to the therapy as follows:

1. Determine the pulse rate. (Count for at least one minute.)

2. Determine the respiratory rate. (Count for at least one minute.)

3. Observe respiration to identify any abnormalities in the breathing pattern.

4. Note any abnormalities in the patient's appearance or behavior.

K. **_Conclude Procedure._** Complete the following tasks:

1. Place the patient in a comfortable position.

2. Assure that the call bell and bedside table are within the patient's reach.

3. Ask if the patient has any needs.

4. Answer any questions as effectively as possible.

L. **_Record Results._** Document the therapy as follows:

1. Record the following data on the patient's chart:

   - Date
   - Time
   - Therapy administered; indicate delivery device and gas-flow rate or FIO_2
   - Pulse rate
   - Respiratory rate
   - Abnormal patient characteristics
   - Therapy-related patient complaints

2. Sign the patient's chart (first initial and full last name).

M. **_Report Observations._** Report the following information:

1. Report any significant adverse changes in the patient's condition to the nurse or physician whenever observed.

2. Following the procedure, inform the appropriate personnel of:

   - Patient requests
   - Patient complaints
   - Unexpressed patient needs

3. Following procedure, report to the nurse or physician:

   - Any non-critical adverse reactions to the therapy
   - Other pertinent observations of the patient's condition

Evaluation of Oxygen Administration Procedures

The following definitions are provided for use whenever oxygen administration procedures are evaluated. In order for performance of the procedures to be considered acceptable, all Essential Tasks are to be performed according to the accompanying Evaluation Criteria. Any deviation from the following task sequence or criteria must be approved by the evaluator.

CPE 9.1 Oxygen Therapy		
Performance	**Essential Tasks**	**Evaluation Criteria**
A. Check Order	See SSE 3.1	See SSE 3.1
B. Review Chart	See SSE 3.2	See SSE 3.2
C. Maintain Asepsis	See SSE 1.2	See SSE 1.2
D. Obtain Equipment	1. Obtains the following equipment and supplies: • Oxygen flowmeter • Humidifier • Sterile water • Oxygen supply tubing • Prescribed delivery device • "No Smoking" signs	a. Correct equipment obtained
E. Assemble Equipment	1. Prepares equipment as follows: • Fills humidifier • Assembles humidifier, tubing, tubing, and flowmeter	a. Sterile water used b. Humidifier filled c. Assembled according to order and **SOP**
F. Test Equipment	1. Tests for: • Functioning of alarm • Leaks in system	a. Tested according to **SOP** b. Leaks remedied c. Defective equipment replaced
G. Confirm Patient	See SSE 3.3	See SSE 3.3

CPE 9.1
Oxygen Therapy (continued)

Performance	Essential Tasks	Evaluation Criteria
H. Inform Patient	See SSE 4.1	See SSE 4.1
I. Implement Procedure	1. Posts "No Smoking" signs	a. Posted on the door b. Posted above bed or in other suitable location
	2. Administers therapy	a. Correct flow rate used b. Delivery device attached correctly c. If bag used, maintained at least 1/3 full
J. Monitor Patient	1. Determines: • Pulse rate • Respiratory rate	a. Counted for at least one (1) minute
	2. Observes: • Respiratory pattern • Patient appearance	a. Any abnormalities identified
K. Conclude Procedure	1. Replaces call bell and bedside table	a. Placed within patient's reach
	2. Tends to patient needs	a. Comfortable position assured b. Patient asked regarding other needs c. Patient questions answered effectively
L. Record Results	See SSE 3.4	See SSE 3.4
M. Report Observations	See SSE 4.3	See SSE 4.3

Module 10.0

Aerosol Administration

Patients are administered aerosol therapy to treat or prevent a humidity deficit in the respiratory system. The procedure involves the generation and delivery of tiny particles of water by means of an aerosol nebulizer. An aerosol can also be used to assist in the production of a sputum specimen and to deliver certain medications. This module addresses the performance of aerosol therapy, sputum induction, and the delivery of aerosol medication.

Objectives

Upon completion of this module, you will be able to:

1. List and explain the conditions that indicate the need for aerosol administration.

2. List and describe the potential hazards associated with aerosol administration.

3. Explain the relationship between flow rate and oxygen concentration when using a jet nebulizer.

4. Assemble and test all equipment necessary for the delivery of aerosol therapy.

5. Administer aerosol therapy according to the procedure prescribed for a patient.

6. Administer aerosol by means of a metered dose inhaler (MDI).

7. Obtain a sputum specimen according to the procedure prescribed for a patient.

8. Administer aerosol medication according to the procedure prescribed for a patient.

Air in the alveoli is saturated with water vapor. The sources of this water vapor are: (1) the humidity already present in inspired air and (2) the moisture added as the air passes through the airway. In situations where the water vapor provided by these two sources is inadequate, additional humidity can be added to the inspired air by means of a humidifier or an aerosol generator. A humidifier is most commonly used to prevent a humidity deficit by adding water vapor to a gas as it is delivered to a patient. Although aerosol generators are sometimes used for this same purpose, they are used more frequently for the therapeutic effects associated with the deposition of very fine droplets of liquid water into the respiratory tract.

Equipment for Aerosol Administration

An aerosol consists of tiny liquid particles suspended in a gas. To produce an aerosol, a special piece of equipment known as a nebulizer is needed. The two most common aerosol generators are the jet and ultrasonic nebulizers. In this section, these two types of nebulizers and the associated equipment used to generate an aerosol are briefly described. In addition, the procedures for assembling and testing the equipment for aerosol administration are presented.

Jet Nebulizers

The most common method of producing an aerosol for use in respiratory therapy is by means of a jet nebulizer. This device utilizes a high-velocity gas flow to generate aerosol particles from a water reservoir by means of the Bernoulli effect. Depending on the needs of the patient, a source gas of either air or oxygen may be used.

The concentration of supplemental oxygen delivered by a jet nebulizer can be regulated by mixing room air with a source of pure oxygen. The mixing is accomplished by means of an air dilutor located at the top of the nebulizer. When the air dilutor is closed, 100% oxygen will be delivered. Opening the air dilutor causes room air to be entrained and mixed with the oxygen source. By adjusting the volume of air entrained, a prescribed concentration of gas can be delivered to the patient.

It should be apparent that the entrainment of room air will cause an increase in the total volume of gas delivered by a jet nebulizer. For this reason, the air dilutor can be used to regulate the total flow of gas delivered as well as to control the concentration of oxygen. For the same reason, the total volume of gas will also be affected any time the air dilutor is used to regulate a patient's oxygen concentration. This means that special precautions may be necessary to ensure adequate gas flow whenever a jet nebulizer is used to provide oxygen in high concentrations.

It is important that the total volume of gas delivered by a nebulizer be sufficient to meet the patient's demand. If the total gas flow is inadequate, room air will enter around the sides of the mask. Because this air does not pass through the nebulizer, it will reduce the particle concentration of the aerosol delivered. To assure an adequate flow rate to meet the inspiratory demand of the patient, a second flowmeter and nebulizer may need to be added to the system.

Ultrasonic Nebulizers

Another device used to administer aerosol therapy is the ultrasonic nebulizer. This device employs sound waves to disperse water particles into the gas medium. Ultrasonic nebulizers ordinarily produce a smaller particle size and higher particle concentration than jet nebulizers. Consequently, they are very effective cough stimulators and are often used for sputum induction. Because of the particle size and concentration, however, the aerosol can also be more hazardous for the patient. For this reason, ultrasonic nebulizers are more frequently used for intermittent therapy than for continuous therapy.

Either a jet nebulizer, metered dose inhaler, or an ultrasonic nebulizer can be prescribed for aerosol therapy. The device used depends upon the condition of the patient and the preference of the physician. Likewise, either type of aerosol generator can be used for sputum induction, but an ultrasonic nebulizer is used more frequently for this procedure. Because either type of nebulizer can be used for either of the two forms of therapy, **Clinical Procedures 10.1 and 10.2** include both types of equipment. When performing these procedures, you should follow the steps for obtaining, assembling, and testing the equipment as prescribed.

Jet Medication Nebulizers

For the unassisted delivery of aerosol medications, a jet medication nebulizer is ordinarily used. This special type of jet nebulizer is characterized by its small size. The use of an ordinary jet nebulizer to deliver medications would require large quantities of the drug in order to maintain the desired concentration in the aerosol. Since most of the drugs delivered as an aerosol are quite expensive, the jet medication nebulizer is more cost-effective.

Metered Dose Inhaler

For many patients, the metered dose inhaler (MDI) is an efficient and cost-effective method of delivering aerosolized medications. In order to use the MDI properly, the patient must be capable of coordinating his or her respiratory efforts and have the hand strength to compress the mechanical device simultaneously. The MDI is the most cost-effective means of delivering aerosol to the patient who is able to perform the required functions.

Administration Technique

The effectiveness of aerosol therapy is greatly influenced by the technique of administration. To obtain the desired penetration and deposition of aerosol particles, breathing instructions should be given to the patient. Slow, deep, diaphragmatic breathing through the mouth provides the most effective results. In addition, a brief pause at the end of inspiration is desirable.

The patient should be routinely monitored during the administration of aerosol therapy. Adverse responses to the aerosol may have important implications for the therapy. Consequently, any changes in the patient's vital signs or appearance should be noted and brought to the attention of the physician.

Clinical Procedure 10.1
Aerosol Therapy

The primary purpose of aerosol therapy is to deliver tiny droplets of water and/or drugs throughout the respiratory system. Ordinarily, it is desirable to achieve sufficient penetration of the system for deposition to occur in all parts of the lower airway, including the alveoli. The principal factors influencing where the deposition takes place are the size and concentration of the particles in the aerosol.

Indications for Aerosol Therapy

Although you will only administer aerosol therapy when ordered by the physician, you should be familiar with the conditions that indicate a need for the procedure. The primary indications for aerosol therapy are:

1. Prevention of a humidity deficit resulting from the inspiration of a dry gas.

2. Dehydration of nasal and pulmonary mucosa resulting from the inspiration of a dry gas, as seen in postsurgical patients.

3. Presence of a humidity deficit resulting from inspired air bypassing the upper airway during the use of an artificial airway.

4. Presence of thick, retained secretions due to conditions such as chronic bronchitis or cystic fibrosis.

Potential Hazards of Aerosol Therapy

Aerosol therapy can have detrimental as well as therapeutic effects on the patient. Potential hazards of aerosol therapy include:

1. Airway obstruction from the swelling of dried, retained secretions.

2. Bronchospasm caused by the inhalation of fine aerosol particles.

3. Fluid overload, especially in infants receiving continuous aerosol therapy.

Procedure for Aerosol Therapy

It is recommended that the following procedure be used for administering aerosol therapy prescribed for a patient:

A. *Check Order.* Verify the physician's order as follows:

1. Compare the requisition with the physician's order to ensure that no discrepancies exist.

2. Review the order to ensure that the following are prescribed:

    - Type of nebulizer to be used
    - FIO_2 (if other than room air)
    - Solution to be used
    - Frequency of therapy
    - Duration of therapy

3. If any part of the order is unfamiliar, question its accuracy.

B. *Review Chart.* Use the following procedure to review the patient's chart:

1. On the patient's chart, identify all pertinent data in the following areas:

    - History and physical
    - Admitting diagnosis
    - Progress notes
    - Blood gas analysis
    - Chest x-rays

2. Based on the patient data, identify the following:

    - Conditions that indicate the need for aerosol therapy
    - Potential hazards of aerosol therapy for the patient

C. *Maintain Asepsis.* While performing the remainder of this procedure, you are expected to maintain aseptic conditions according to the procedure described in **SSE 1.2**. This includes using universal precautions and washing your hands:

- Before obtaining equipment
- Following performance of step **K. Conclude Procedure**
- Anytime during the procedure that contamination is suspected

Note: The next three steps (D through F) will vary according to the type of equipment ordered. Proceed with the set of steps which corresponds with the equipment prescribed for the patient.

• • • • • • • • •

Jet Nebulizer

D.   *Obtain Equipment.* Collect the following equipment and supplies:

- Jet nebulizer
- Flowmeter(s)
- Mainstream tubing
- Delivery device
- Prescribed solution
- Oxygen analyzer (if indicated)
- "No Smoking" signs (if supplemental oxygen is ordered)
- Stethoscope

E.   *Assemble Equipment.* Prepare the equipment for use as follows:

1. Fill the nebulizer to the fill line with solution.

2. Connect the mainstream tubing to the nebulizer.

3. Attach the other end of the mainstream tubing to the aerosol delivery device.

4. Connect the flowmeter to the gas inlet of the nebulizer.

F.   *Test Equipment.* Test the aerosol delivery equipment as follows:

1. Connect the flowmeter to the correct gas source.

2. Adjust the flowmeter to 10 liters per minute.

3. If a fine mist is absent, tighten all connections and press the jet cleaner button several times.

4. If a fine mist is still absent:

   a. Label the nebulizer as "defective" and replace it.
   b. Reassemble and retest the new equipment.

• • • • • • • •

Ultrasonic Nebulizer

D. *Obtain Equipment.* Collect the following equipment and supplies:

- Ultrasonic nebulizer
- Couplant and cover
- Power source (flowmeter and supply tubing or ultrasonic blower)
- Mainstream tubing
- Delivery device
- Prescribed solution
- Oxygen analyzer (if indicated)
- "No Smoking" signs (if supplemental oxygen is ordered)
- Stethoscope

E. *Assemble Equipment.* Prepare the equipment for use as follows:

1. Place the couplant inside the ultrasonic chamber.

2. Fill the ultrasonic chamber to the appropriate level with water.

3. Cover the couplant and ultrasonic chamber with the couplant cover.

4. Attach the mainstream tubing to the couplant elbow.

5. Attach the other end of the mainstream tubing to the delivery device.

6. Attach the power source to the other couplant elbow.

7. Fill the couplant with the prescribed solution.

F. *Test Equipment.* Test the aerosol delivery equipment as follows:

1. Plug the ultrasonic nebulizer cord into an electrical outlet.

2. Turn on the ultrasonic nebulizer.

3. Adjust the frequency as necessary to produce a fine mist.

4. If a fine mist is absent:

   a. Ensure that the diaphragm is in contact with the transducer.
   b. Check for a film on the diaphragm.
   c. Adjust or clean the diaphragm.

5. If a fine mist is still absent:

   a. Label the nebulizer as "defective" and replace it.
   b. Reassemble and retest the new equipment.

· · · · · · · ·

G. Confirm Patient. Ensure that the procedure is performed with the correct patient as follows:

1. Match the information on the order with the following:

   • Room number
   • Name on the door or bed
   • Name on the wristband

2. Greet the patient by name (in a questioning manner if unknown).

3. Resolve any discrepancies in the patient identification information by conferring with the nursing staff.

H. Inform Patient. Interact with the patient as follows:

1. Introduce yourself by name and department (if not already acquainted).

2. Tell the patient what procedure is to be performed.

3. Explain the procedure by describing:

   • Why it is to be performed
   • How it will be performed
   • What the patient is expected to do
   • What you will be doing
   • How frequently it will be performed

4. Explain the fire hazards associated with the use of oxygen and caution the patient against smoking.

I. Implement Procedure. Perform the following tasks:

1. If supplemental oxygen is ordered, post "No Smoking" signs above the bed and on the door.

2. Position the patient in an upright position (45 to 90° angle).

3. Administer aerosol therapy as follows:

    a. Adjust the flowmeter to the prescribed gas flow rate.
    b. Attach the aerosol delivery device to the patient.
    c. Ensure that the delivery device fits comfortably.
    d. If a specific concentration of supplemental oxygen is ordered, analyze the gas and adjust the equipment as necessary to establish the prescribed FIO_2.

4. Coach the patient to breathe in the following manner:

   - Diaphragmatically
   - Through the mouth
   - Slowly and deeply
   - Pause at end-inspiration, maintaining an I:E ratio of at least 1:2

J. *Monitor Patient.* Determine the patient's response to therapy as follows:

1. Determine the pulse rate. (Count for at least one minute.)

2. Determine the respiratory rate. (Count for at least one minute.)

3. Observe respirations to identify any abnormalities in the breathing pattern.

4. Auscultate the patient's chest according to the procedure described in **SSE 2.2.**

5. Note any abnormalities in the patient's appearance or behavior.

K. *Conclude Procedure.* Complete the following tasks:

1. Place the patient in a comfortable position.

2. Assure that the call bell and bedside table are within the patient's reach.

3. Ask if the patient has any needs.

4. Answer any questions as effectively as possible.

5. Unplug and cover all equipment and move it away from the patient's bed (or remove it from the room).

L. Record Results. Document the therapy as follows:

   1. Record the following data on the patient's chart:

- Date
- Time
- Therapy administered; indicate delivery device, gas flow rate, and/or FIO_2
- Pulse rate
- Respiratory rate
- Abnormal patient characteristics
- Therapy-related patient complaints

   2. Sign the patient's chart (first initial and full last name).

M. Report Observations. Report the following information:

   1. Report any significant adverse changes in the patient's condition to the nurse or physician whenever observed.

   2. Following the procedure, inform the appropriate personnel of:

- Patient requests
- Patient complaints
- Unexpressed patient needs

   3. Following the procedure, report to the nurse or physician:

- Any non-critical adverse reactions to the therapy
- Other pertinent observations of the patient's condition

Clinical Procedure 10.2
Sputum Induction

Cooperative, alert patients are sometimes unable to produce a sputum specimen by unassisted cough. In such cases, it may be necessary to assist the patient with aerosol therapy. For sputum induction, sterile water or hypertonic saline solutions are generally used in the nebulizer. Both are more effective in stimulating a cough than normal saline because they are more irritating.

In most instances, sputum induction is not a hazardous procedure. Occasionally, however, a patient may experience bronchospasm or airway obstruction from the rapid mobilization of secretions. When this happens, the aerosol delivery should be discontinued, the airway cleared, and the physician notified.

In preparation for sputum induction, the patient should be instructed to perform the necessary activities to remove any debris present in the nasal and oropharyngeal cavity. These include blowing the nose, brushing the teeth, and gargling with normal saline.

Sputum should be collected in a sterile cup. Once a sufficient quantity (1 cc or more) is collected, it should be sent to the laboratory immediately. A "sputum" specimen should be discarded if it contains food particles, consists only of saliva, or is not examined while fresh.

Procedure for Sputum Induction

Whenever a respiratory care order prescribes the administration of an aerosol for the purpose of sputum induction, the following procedure is suggested:

A. *Check Order.* Verify the physician's order as follows:

1. Compare the requisition with the physician's order to ensure that no discrepancies exist.

2. Review the order to ensure that the following are prescribed:

   - Type of nebulizer to be used
   - FIO_2
   - Solution to be used
   - Frequency of therapy
   - Duration of therapy

3. If any part of the order is unfamiliar, question its accuracy.

B. ***Review Chart.*** Use the following procedure to review the patient's chart:

1. On the patient's chart, identify all pertinent data in the following areas:

   - History and physical
   - Admitting diagnosis
   - Progress notes
   - Blood gas analysis
   - Chest x-rays

2. Based on the patient data, identify the following:

   - Conditions that indicate the need for sputum induction
   - Potential hazards of sputum induction for the patient

C. ***Maintain Asepsis.*** While performing the remainder of this procedure, you are expected to maintain aseptic conditions according to the procedure described in **SSE 1.2**. This includes following universal precautions and washing your hands:

- Before obtaining equipment
- Following performance of step ***N. Conclude Procedure***
- Anytime during the procedure that contamination is suspected

Note: The next three steps (D through F) will vary according to the type of equipment ordered. Proceed with the set of steps that corresponds with the equipment prescribed for the patient.

• • • • • • • •

Jet Nubulizer

D. ***Obtain Equipment.*** Collect the following equipment and supplies:

- Jet nebulizer
- Flowmeter(s)
- Mainstream tubing
- Delivery device
- Prescribed solution
- Oxygen analyzer (if indicated)
- "No Smoking" signs (if supplemental oxygen is ordered)
- Stethoscope

E. ***Assemble Equipment.*** Prepare the equipment for use as follows:

1. Fill the nebulizer to the fill line with solution.

2. Connect the mainstream tubing to the nebulizer.

3. Attach the other end of the mainstream tubing to the aerosol delivery device.

4. Connect the flowmeter to the gas inlet of the nebulizer.

F. ***Test Equipment.*** Test the aerosol delivery equipment as follows:

1. Connect the flowmeter to the correct gas source.

2. Adjust the flowmeter to 10 liters per minute.

3. If a fine mist is absent, tighten all connections and press the jet cleaner button several times.

4. If a fine mist is still absent:

   a. Label the nebulizer as "defective" and replace it.
   b. Reassemble and retest the new equipment.

• • • • • • • •

Ultrasonic Nebulizer

D. ***Obtain Equipment.*** Collect the following equipment and supplies:

- Ultrasonic nebulizer
- Couplant and cover
- Power source (flowmeter and supply tubing or ultrasonic blower)
- Mainstream tubing
- Delivery device
- Prescribed solution
- Oxygen analyzer (if indicated)
- "No Smoking" signs (if supplemental oxygen is ordered)
- Stethoscope

E. ***Assemble Equipment.*** Prepare the equipment for use as follows:

1. Place the couplant inside the ultrasonic chamber.

2. Fill the ultrasonic chamber to the appropriate level with water.

3. Cover the couplant and ultrasonic chamber with the couplant cover.

4. Attach the mainstream tubing to the couplant elbow.

5. Attach the other end of the mainstream tubing to the delivery device.

6. Attach the power source to the other couplant elbow.

7. Fill the couplant with the prescribed solution.

F. **Test Equipment.** Test the aerosol delivery equipment as follows:

1. Plug the ultrasonic nebulizer cord into an electrical outlet.

2. Turn on the ultrasonic nebulizer.

3. Adjust the frequency as necessary to produce a fine mist.

4. If a fine mist is absent:

   a. Ensure that the diaphragm is in contact with the transducer.
   b. Check for a film on the diaphragm.
   c. Adjust or clean the diaphragm.

5. If a fine mist is still absent:

   a. Label the nebulizer as "defective" and replace it.
   b. Reassemble and retest the new equipment.

• • • • • • • •

G. **Confirm Patient.** Ensure that the procedure is performed with the correct patient as follows:

1. Match the information on the order with the following:

   • Room number
   • Name on the door or bed
   • Name on the wristband

2. Greet the patient by name (in a questioning manner if unknown).

3. Resolve any discrepancies in the patient identification information by conferring with the nursing staff.

H. **_Inform Patient._** Interact with the patient as follows:

1. Introduce yourself by name and department (if not already acquainted).

2. Tell the patient what procedure is to be performed.

3. Explain the procedure by describing:

   - Why it is to be performed
   - How it will be performed
   - What the patient is expected to do
   - What you will be doing
   - How frequently it will be performed

I. **_Ensure Hygiene._** Instruct the patient to:

1. Perform any of the following activities necessary to remove any debris present in the nasal or oropharyngeal airway:

   - Blow the nose
   - Brush the teeth
   - Gargle with normal saline

J. **_Implement Procedure._** Perform the following tasks:

1. If supplemental oxygen is ordered, post "No Smoking" signs above the bed and on the door.

2. Position the patient in an upright position (45 to 90° angle).

3. Administer aerosol as follows:

   a. Adjust the flowmeter to the prescribed gas-flow rate.
   b. Attach the aerosol delivery device to the patient.
   c. Ensure that the delivery device fits comfortably.
   d. If a specific concentration of supplemental oxygen is ordered, analyze the gas and adjust the equipment as necessary to establish the prescribed FIO_2.

4. Coach the patient to breathe in the following manner:

   - Diaphragmatically
   - Through the mouth
   - Slowly and deeply
   - Pause at end-inspiration, maintaining an I:E ratio of at least 1:2

K. *Monitor Patient.* Determine the patient's response to therapy as follows:

1. Determine the pulse rate. (Count for at least one minute.)

2. Determine the respiratory rate. (Count for at least one minute.)

3. Observe respirations to identify any abnormalities in the breathing pattern.

4. Auscultate the patient's chest according to the procedure described in **SSE 2.2.**

5. Note any abnormalities in the patient's appearance or behavior.

L. *Coach Coughing.* Assist the patient in coughing as follows:

1. Encourage the patient to cough:

   • Immediately following aerosol administration
   • As needed during the following procedure to achieve an appropriate cough

2. Assist the patient by performing the following as needed:

   • Percussion
   • Vibration
   • Tussive squeeze
   • Localized breathing coaching

M. *Collect Sputum.* Using a sterile container:

1. Obtain a sufficient quantity of sputum (at least 1 cc).

2. Label the container to indicate:

   • Patient name
   • Room number
   • Contents
   • Date
   • Time

N. *Conclude Procedure.* Complete the following tasks:

1. Place the patient in a comfortable position.

2. Assure that the call bell and bedside table are within the patient's reach.

3. Ask if the patient has any needs.

4. Answer any questions as effectively as possible.

5. Unplug and cover all equipment and move it away from the patient's bed (or remove it from the room).

O. ***Record Results.*** Document the therapy as follows:

1. Record the following data on the patient's chart:

   • Date
   • Time
   • Therapy administered; indicate delivery device, gas flow rate, and/or FIO_2
   • Pulse rate
   • Respiratory rate
   • Abnormal patient characteristics
   • Therapy-related patient complaints
   • Volume, color, and consistency of sputum

2. Sign the patient's chart (first initial and full last name).

P. ***Report Observations.*** Report the following information:

1. Report any significant adverse changes in the patient's condition to the nurse or physician whenever observed.

2. Following the procedure, inform the appropriate personnel of:

   • Patient requests
   • Patient complaints
   • Unexpressed patient needs

3. Following the procedure, report to the nurse or physician:

   • Any noncritical adverse reactions to the therapy
   • Other pertinent observations of the patient's condition

Q. ***Dispense Specimen.*** Following hospital protocol:

1. Deliver the sputum specimen to the proper laboratory for analysis.

Clinical Procedure 10.3
Aerosol Medication Therapy

Certain drugs are most effective when administered directly into the airway. For example, bronchodilators have a faster response time when administered as an aerosol rather than systemically. Aerosolized medications are often delivered to liquefy and help remove retained secretions.

The administration of aerosol medications is accompanied by the same hazards that are associated with aerosol therapy. In addition, aerosol medications introduce the risk of adverse drug reactions. Possible side effects include increased heart rate, cardiac arrhythmia, nervousness, and bronchospasm. Before administering any drug, its possible side effects should be noted. If evidence of any of these side effects is detected, the therapy should be discontinued and the physician notified.

Procedure for Aerosol Medication Delivery

The following procedure is provided for use when delivering medications by means of an aerosol generator:

A. **Check Order.** Verify the physician's order as follows:

   1. Compare the requisition with the physician's order to ensure that no discrepancies exist.

   2. Review the order to ensure that the following are prescribed:

     • FIO_2
     • Medication to be used
     • Frequency of therapy
     • Duration of therapy

   3. If any part of the order is unfamiliar, question its accuracy.

B. **Review Chart.** Use the following procedure to review the patient's chart:

   1. On the patient's chart, identify all pertinent data in the following areas:

     • History and physical
     • Admitting diagnosis

- Progress notes
- Blood gas analysis
- Chest x-rays

2. Based on the patient data, identify the following:

   - Conditions that indicate the need for aerosol medication delivery
   - Potential hazards of aerosol medication delivery for the patient

C. *Maintain Asepsis.* While performing the remainder of this procedure, you are expected to maintain aseptic conditions according to the procedure described in **SSE 1.2.** This includes following universal precautions and washing your hands:

   - Before obtaining equipment
   - Following performance of step **K. Conclude Procedure**
   - Anytime during the procedure that contamination is suspected

D. *Obtain Equipment.* Collect the following equipment and supplies:

   - Flowmeter or air compressor
   - Miniature nebulizer
   - Supply tubing
   - Prescribed medication
   - Stethoscope

E. *Assemble Equipment.* Prepare the equipment for use as follows:

   1. Connect the supply tubing to the nebulizer.

   2. Attach the other end of the supply tubing to the flowmeter.

   3. Insert the prescribed medication into the nebulizer.

F. *Test Equipment.* Test the aerosol medication delivery equipment as follows:

   1. Connect the flowmeter to the correct gas source.

   2. Turn on the flowmeter.

   3. If a fine mist is absent, tighten all connections and adjust the jets, if applicable.

   4. If a fine mist is still absent:

      a. Label the nebulizer as "defective" and replace it.
      b. Reassemble and retest the new equipment.

G. ***Confirm Patient.*** Ensure that the procedure is performed with the correct patient as follows:

1. Match the information on the order with the following:

   • Room number
   • Name on the door or bed
   • Name on the wristband

2. Greet the patient by name (in a questioning manner if unknown).

3. Resolve any discrepancies in the patient identification information by conferring with the nursing staff.

H. ***Inform Patient.*** Interact with the patient as follows:

1. Introduce yourself by name and department (if not already acquainted).

2. Tell the patient what procedure is to be performed.

3. Explain the procedure by describing:

   • Why it is to be performed
   • How it will be performed
   • What the patient is expected to do
   • What you will be doing
   • How frequently it will be performed

I. ***Implement Procedure.*** Perform the following tasks:

1. Position the patient in an upright position (45 to 90° angle).

2. Administer the aerosol medication as follows:

   a. Turn on the flowmeter.
   b. Attach the aerosol medication delivery device to the patient.
   c. Ensure that the delivery device fits comfortably.

3. Coach the patient to breathe in the following manner:

   • Diaphragmatically
   • Through the mouth
   • Slowly and deeply
   • Pause at end-inspiration, maintaining an I:E ratio of at least 1:2

Notes

J. **Monitor Patient.** Determine the patient's response to therapy as follows:

1. Determine the pulse rate. (Count for at least one minute.)

2. Determine the respiratory rate. (Count for at least one minute.)

3. Observe respirations to identify any abnormalities in the breathing pattern.

4. Auscultate the patient's chest according to the procedure described in **SSE 2.2.**

5. Note any abnormalities in the patient's appearance or behavior.

K. **Conclude Procedure.** Complete the following tasks:

1. Place the patient in a comfortable position.

2. Assure that the call bell and bedside table are within the patient's reach.

3. Ask if the patient has any needs.

4. Answer any questions as effectively as possible.

5. Unplug and cover all equipment and move it away from the patient's bed (or remove it from the room).

L. **Record Results.** Document the therapy as follows:

1. Record the following data on the patient's chart:

   - Aerosol medication administered
   - Pulse rate
   - Respiratory rate
   - Volume, color, and consistency of sputum
   - Abnormal patient characteristics
   - Therapy-related patient complaints

2. Sign the patient's chart (first initial and full last name).

M. **Report Observations.** Report the following information:

1. Report any significant adverse changes in the patient's condition to the nurse or physician whenever observed.

2. Following the procedure, inform the appropriate personnel of:

- Patient requests
- Patient complaints
- Unexpressed patient needs

3. Following the procedure, report to the nurse or physician:

- Any non-critical adverse reactions to the therapy
- Other pertinent observations of the patient's condition

Clinical Procedure 10.4
Metered Dose Inhaler

The metered dose inhaler (MDI) is a cost-effective alternative to the jet nebulizer for the delivery of aerosol medication. The MDI is a device manufactured by pharmaceutical companies that contains pre-measured doses of aerosolized drugs. To administer the drug, the patient holds the inhaler and compresses the medication chamber while inspiring and inhales the prescribed dose of medication. Often, three or more puffs of the medication are required to meet the prescribed dose.

Indications

The metered dose inhaler is indicated for the self-sufficient patient who requires certain types of aerosolized medications. The patient who will require the delivery of an aerosol medication after leaving the hospital is often converted to a metered dose inhaler before being discharged. The MDI is sometimes prescribed for patients during their stay in the hospital in order to reduce the cost of bedside treatment administered by a respiratory therapist. Whenever a patient is expected to use an MDI, instruction in its use must be provided by a trained health care professional.

Potential Hazards

All of the hazards associated with the delivery of aerosol medication by means of a nebulizer apply to the metered dose inhaler. Possible adverse drug reactions include: Increased heart rate, cardiac arrhythmias, nervousness, and bronchospasm. In addition, the possible side effects of any specific drug should be noted before it is administered. If evidence of any of these side effects is detected, therapy should be discontinued and the physician notified.

One of the biggest problems with MDI therapy is the inability of the patient to perform the procedure correctly. The patient must have sufficient muscle strength in the hands to compress the medication chamber completely. Coordination is involved to begin inspiration in conjunction with compression of the chamber. Special devices or chambers are available to prevent the loss of medication should the patient fail to coordinate properly.

Procedure for Administering Metered Dose Inhaler

The following procedure is provided for use when delivering medications by means of a metered dose inhaler:

A. **Check Order.** Verify the physician's order as follows:

1. Compare the requisition with the physician's order to ensure that no discrepancies exist.

2. Review the order to ensure that the following are prescribed:

    • Medication to be used
    • Frequency of therapy
    • Duration of therapy
    • Any special devices or chambers required

B. **Review Chart.** Use the following procedure to review the patient's chart:

1. On the patient's chart, identify all pertinent data in the following areas:

    • History and physical
    • Admitting diagnosis
    • Progress notes
    • Blood gas analysis
    • Chest X-rays

2. Based on the patient data, identify the following:

    • Conditions that indicate the need for metered dose inhaler delivery
    • Potential hazards of aerosol medication delivery for the patient

C. **Maintain Asepsis.** While performing the remainder of this procedure, you are expected to maintain aseptic conditions according to the procedures described in **SSE 1.2.** This includes the use of universal precautions and handwashing. Hands should be washed:

    • Before obtaining equipment
    • Following performance of step *J. Conclude Procedure*
    • Anytime during the procedure that contamination is suspected.

D. *Obtain Equipment.* Collect the following equipment and supplies:

- Metered Dose Inhaler (as prescribed)
- Any special devices or chambers (as applicable)
- Stethoscope

E. *Assemble Equipment.* Prepare the equipment for use as follows:

1. Shake the inhaler to mix the medications.

2. Remove the cap and attach the mouthpiece.

3. If a chamber is ordered, attach the device to the mouthpiece.

F. *Confirm Patient.* Ensure that the procedure is performed on the correct patient as follows:

1. Match the information on the order with the following:

    - Room number
    - Name on the door or bed
    - Name on the wristband

2. Greet the patient by name (in a questioning manner if unknown).

3. Resolve any discrepancies in the patient identification information by conferring with the nursing staff.

G. *Inform Patient.* Interact with the patient as follows:

1. Introduce yourself by name and department (if not already acquainted).

2. Tell the patient what procedure is to be performed.

3. Explain the procedure by describing:

    - Why it is to be performed
    - How it will be performed
    - What the patient is expected to do
    - What you will be doing
    - How frequently it will be performed

H. *Implement Procedure.* Perform the following tasks:

1. Position the patient in an upright position (45 to 90 ° angle).

2. Instruct the patient as follows:

   a. Grasp the MDI medication chamber between the thumb and first two fingers with the thumb on the bottom of the chamber.

   b. Hold the mouthpiece of the medication chamber (or additional chamber device if ordered) in front of the mouth with the lips around the mouthpiece but not closed on it.

   c. If the patient has difficulty holding the device without closing the lips, instruct him/her to rest the mouthpiece on the lower lip for balance.

   d. Exhale completely. Begin to inhale deeply through the mouth and immediately compress the medication chamber between the thumb and fingers to release the medication.

   e. Following complete inhalation, hold his/her breath for 5 to 10 seconds.

   f. If an additional chamber was used, inhale from the device again, without compressing the medication chamber, to ensure complete aerosol delivery.

   g. Repeat the process until the prescribed duration is accomplished.

I. *Monitor Patient.* Determine the patient's response to the therapy as follows:

1. Determine the pulse rate. (Count for at least one minute).

2. Determine the respiratory rate. (Count for at least one minute).

3. Observe respirations to identify any abnormalities in the breathing pattern.

4. Auscultate the patient's chest according to the procedure described in **SSE 2.2.**

5. Note any abnormalities in the patient's appearance or behavior.

J. *Conclude Procedure.* Complete the following tasks:

1. Place the patient in a comfortable position.

2. Assure that the call bell and bedside table are within the patient's reach.

3. Ask if the patient has any needs.

4. Answer any questions as effectively as possible.

K. *Record Results.* Record the following data on the laboratory data form and on the patient's chart as required:

- Patient name
- Room number
- Aerosol medication delivered
- Pulse rate
- Respiratory rate
- Breath sounds
- Volume, color and consistence of sputum
- Any adverse patient reactions
- Therapy-related patient complaints

L. *Report Observations.* Report the following information:

1. Report any significant adverse changes in the patient's condition to the nurse or physician.

2. Following the procedure, inform the appropriate personnel of:

- Patient requests
- Patient complaints
- Unexpressed patient needs

3. Following the procedure, report to the nurse or physician:

- Any non-critical adverse reactions to the therapy
- Other pertinent observations of the patient's condition

Evaluation of Aerosol Administration Procedures

The following definitions are provided for use whenever the respective Aerosol Administration Procedures are evaluated. In order for performance of the procedures to be considered acceptable, all Essential Tasks must be performed according to the accompanying Evaluation Criteria. Any deviation from the following sequence or criteria for performing the Essential Tasks must be approved by the evaluator.

	CPE 10.1 Aerosol Therapy	
Performance	**Essential Tasks**	**Evaluation Criteria**
A. Check Order	See SSE 3.1	See SSE 3.1
B. Review Chart	See SSE 3.2	See SSE 3.2
C. Maintain Asepsis	See SSE 1.2	See SSE 1.2
D. Obtain Equipment	1. Obtains the following equipment and supplies: • Nebulizer (jet or ultrasonic) • Couplant and cover (if ultrasonic) • Flowmeter(s) or ultrasonic power source • Mainstream tubing • Delivery device • Prescribed solution • Oxygen analyzer (if required) • "No Smoking" signs (if required) • Stethoscope	a. Correct equipment obtained
E. Assemble Equipment	1. Prepares equipment as follows: • Places couplant inside chamber (if ultrasonic) • Fills nebulizer • Covers couplant and chamber (if ultrasonic)	a. Correct solution used b. Solution added to line c. Assembled according to **SOP** order

CPE 10.1
Aerosol Therapy (continued)

Performance	Essential Tasks	Evaluation Criteria
E. Assemble Equipment (continued)	• Connects nebulizer, delivery device and flowmeter(s) or power source.	
F. Test Equipment	1. Tests for: • Functioning of equipment • Leaks in system	a. Tested according to **SOP** b. Leaks remedied c. Effort made to correct any equipment malfunction d. Fine mist produced
G. Confirm Patient	See **SSE 3.3**	See **SSE 3.3**
H. Inform Patient	See **SSE 4.1**	See **SSE 4.1**
I. Implement Procedure	1. Posts "No Smoking" signs	a. Performed when oxygen is ordered b. Posted on the door c. Posted above bed or in other suitable location
	2. Positions patient	a. Placed in upright position (45-90°)
	3. Administers therapy	a. Correct flow rate used b. Delivery device attached correctly c. Prescribed FIO_2 delivered
	4. Coaches patient to breathe: • Diaphrigmatically • Through mouth • Slowly and deeply • Pause at end-inspiration	a. Clear and accurate instructions provided b. Patient performance encouraged c. Instructions repeated as needed
J. Monitor Patient	1. Determines: • Pulse rate • Respiratory rate	a. Counted for at least one (1) minute

CPE 10.1 Aerosol Therapy (continued)		
Performance	**Essential Tasks**	**Evaluation Criteria**
J. Monitor Patient (continued)	2. Observes: • Respiratory pattern • Patient appearance	a. Any abnormalities identified
	3. Auscultates chest	a. Performed according to **SSE 2.3**
K. Conclude Procedure	1. Restores room to original condition	a. Equipment removed from room or covered and moved to suitable location withing room b. Call bell and bedside table positioned within patient's reach
	2. Tends to patient needs	a. Comfortable position assured b. Patient asked regarding other needs c. Patient questions answered effectively
L. Record Results	See **SSE 3.4**	See **SSE 3.4**
M. Report Observations	See **SSE 4.3**	See **SSE 4.3**

CPE 10.2 Sputum Induction		
Performance	Essential Tasks	Evaluation Criteria
A. Check Order	See SSE 3.1	See SSE 3.1
B. Review Chart	See SSE 3.2	See SSE 3.2
C. Maintain Asepsis	See SSE 1.2	See SSE 1.2
D. Obtain Equipment	1. Obtains the following equipment and supplies: • Nebulizer (jet or ultrasonic) • Couplant and cover (if ultrasonic) • Flowmeter(s) or ultrasonic power source • Mainstream tubing • Delivery device • Prescribed solution • Oxygen analyzer (if required) • "No Smoking" signs (if required) • Stethoscope. • Sputum specimen container.	a. Correct equipment obtained
E. Assemble Equipment	1. Prepares equipment as follows: • Places couplant inside chamber (if ultrasonic). • Fills nebulizer. • Covers couplant and chamber (if ultrasonic). • Connects nebulizer, delivery device and flowmeter(s) or power source	a. Correct solution used b. Solution added to line c. Assembled according to SOP and order
F. Test Equipment	1. Tests for: • Functioning of equipment • Leaks in system	a. Tested according to SOP b. Leaks remedied c. Effort made to correct any equipment malfunction d. Fine mist produced

CPE 10.2
Sputum Induction (continued)

Performance	Essential Tasks	Evaluation Criteria
G. Confirm Patient	See SSE 3.3	See SSE 3.3
H. Inform Patient	See SSE 4.1	See SSE 4.1
I. Ensure Hygiene	1. Instructs patient to: • Blow nose • Brush teeth • Gargle	a. Performed as needed b. Clear and accurate instructions provided c. Patient performance encouraged
J. Implement Procedure	1. Posts "No Smoking" signs	a. Performed when oxygen is ordered b. Posted on the door c. Posted above bed or in other suitable location
	2. Positions patient	a. Placed in upright position (45-90°)
	3. Administers therapy	a. Correct flow rate used b. Delivery device attached correctly c. Prescribed FIO_2 delivered
	4. Coaches patient to breathe: • Diaphragmatically • Through mouth • Slowly and deeply • Pause at end-inspiration	a. Clear and accurate instructions provided b. Patient performance encouraged c. Instructions repeated as needed
K. Monitor Patient	1. Determines: • Pulse rate • Respiratory rate	a. Counted for at least one (1) minute
	2. Observes: • Respiratory pattern • Patient appearance	a. Any abnormalities identified
	3. Auscultates chest	a. Performed according to SSE 2.3

CPE 10.2 Sputum Induction (continued)		
Performance	**Essential Tasks**	**Evaluation Criteria**
L. Coach Coughing	1. Encourages coughing: • After aerosol administration • As needed	a. Clear and accurate instructions provided b. Instructions repeated as needed
	2. Performs the following when needed: • Percussion • Tussive squeeze • Localized breathing coaching.	a. Performed correctly b. Need correctly determined
M. Collect Sputum	1. Obtains sputum specimen	a. At least 1 cc collected b. Container labeled correctly c. Sterility maintained
N. Conclude Procedure	1. Restores room to original condition	a. Equipment removed from room or covered and moved to suitable location within room b. Call bell and bedside table positioned within patient's reach
	2. Tends to patient needs	a. Comfortable position assured b. Patient asked regarding other needs c. Patient questions answered effectively
O. Record Results	See SSE 3.4	See SSE 3.4
P. Report Observations	See SSE 4.3	See SSE 4.3
Q. Dispense Specimen	1. Delivers specimen to laboratory	a. Hospital protocol followed b. Delivered to correct laboratory

CPE 10.3 Aerosol Medication Delivery		
Performance	**Essential Tasks**	**Evaluation Criteria**
A. Check Order	See **SSE 3.1**	See **SSE 3.1**
B. Review Chart	See **SSE 3.2**	See **SSE 3.2**
C. Maintain Asepsis	See **SSE 1.2**	See **SSE 1.2**
D. Obtain Equipment	1. Obtains the following equipment and supplies: • Flowmeter • Miniature nebulizer • Supply tubing • Prescribed medication • Stethoscope	a. Correct equipment obtained
E. Assemble	1. Prepares equipment as follows: • Connects nebulizer, supply tubing and flowmeter. • Inserts medication.	a. Correct medication used b. Correct medication dosage used c. Assembled according to order and **SOP**
F. Test Equipment	1. Tests for: • Functioning of equipment • Leaks in system	a. Tested according to **SOP** b. Leaks remedied c. Effort made to correct any equipment malfunction d. Fine mist produced
G. Confirm Patient	See **SSE 3.3**	See **SSE 3.3**
H. Inform Patient	See **SSE 4.1**	See **SSE 4.1**
I. Implement Procedure	1. Positions patient	a. Placed in upright position (45-90°)

CPE 10.3 Aerosol Medication Delivery (continued)		
Performance	**Essential Tasks**	**Evaluation Criteria**
I. Implement Procedure (continued)	2. Administers therapy	a. Correct flow rate used b. Delivery device attached correctly c. Prescribed FIO_2 delivered
	3. Coaches patient to breathe: • Diaphragmatically • Through mout • Slowly and deeply • Pause at end-inspiration	a. Clear and accurate instructions provided b. Patient performance encouraged c. Instructions repeated as needed
J. Monitor Patient	1. Determines: • Pulse rate • Respiratory rate	a. Counted for at least one (1) minute b. Repeated at 5-minute intervals
	2. Observes: • Respiratory pattern • Patient appearance	a. Any abnormalities identified
	3. Auscultates chest	a. Performed according to **SSE 2.3**
K. Conclude Procedure	1. Restores room to original condition	a. Equipment removed from froom or covered and moved to suitable location within room b. Call bell and bedside table positioned within patient's reach
	2. Tends to patient needs	a. Comfortable position assured b. Patient asked regarding other needs c. Patient questions answered effectively
L. Record Results	See **SSE 3.4**	See **SSE 3.4**
M. Report Observations	See **SSE 4.3**	See **SSE 4.3**

CPE 10.4 Metered Dose Inhaler		
Performance	**Essential Tasks**	**Evaluation Criteria**
A. Check Order	See SSE 3.1	See SSE 3.1
B. Review Chart	See SSE 3.2	See SSE 3.2
C. Maintain Asepsis	See SSE 1.2	See SSE 1.2
D. Obtain Equipment	1. Obtains the following equipment and supplies: • MDI • Special devices (if ordered) • Stethoscope	a. Correct equipment obtained
E. Assemble Equipment	1. Prepares equipment as follows: follows: • Shakes inhaler • Removes cap and attaches mouthpiece • Attaches chamber if ordered	a. Equipment assembled properly and according to prescription
F. Confirm Patient	See SSE 3.3	See SSE 3.3
G. Inform Patient	See SSE 4.1	See SSE 4.1
H. Implement Procedure	1. Positions patient 2. Instructs patient to: a. Grasp MDI between thumb and fingers b. Hold mouthpiece to mouth with lips open c. Secure MDI with lower lip if having difficulty	a. Placed in upright position (45-90°) a. Clear and accurate instructions provided b. Patient performance encouraged c. Instructions repeated as needed

CPE 10.4 Metered Dose Inhaler (continued)		
Performance	**Essential Tasks**	**Evaluation Criteria**
H. Implement Procedure (continued)	d. Exhale completely and then inhale while compressing MDI e. Hold breath for 5 - 10 seconds f. Repeat inspiration without depressing MDI if additional chamber used g. Repeat procedure until prescription is filled	
I. Monitor Patient	1. Determines: • Pulse rate • Respiratory rate 2. Observes: • Respiratory pattern • Patient Appearance 3. Auscultates chest	a. Counted for at least one (1) minute a. Any abnormalities identified a. Performed according to **SSE 2.3**
J. Conclude Procedure	1. Restores room to original condition 2. Tends to patient needs	a. Equipment removed from room or covered and moved to a suitable location in room b. Call bell and bedside table positioned within patient's reach a. Comfortable position assured b. Patient asked regarding other needs c. Patient's questions answered effectively
K. Record Results	See **SSE 3.4**	See **SSE 3.4**
L. Report Observations	See **SSE 4.3**	See **SSE 4.3**

Module 11.0

Lung Expansion Therapy

Breathing patterns of normal individuals are interrupted periodically by spontaneous deep breaths or sighs. It is believed that these sighs assist in maintaining normal pulmonary compliance, work of breathing, and venous admixture by reinflating atelectatic air spaces. Patients who are unable or unwilling to take periodic deep breaths, or who have chronically decreased compliance of the respiratory system, are often assisted in inflating their lungs. The purpose of this module is to present two methods employed for assisting lung expansion, intermittent positive pressure breathing (IPPB) and incentive spirometry.

Objectives

Upon completion of this module, you will be able to:

1. List and explain conditions that indicate the use of incentive spirometry.

2. List and explain conditions that indicate the use of IPPB therapy.

3. List and describe potential hazards associated with IPPB therapy.

4. Administer incentive spirometry to a patient according to the procedure prescribed.

5. Administer IPPB therapy to a patient according to the procedure prescribed.

It is well documented that patients who breathe at a low constant tidal volume have a tendency toward decreased pulmonary compliance, increased work of breathing and hypoxemia resulting from ventilation-perfusion mismatch. It is believed that the reversal of these conditions may help prevent subsequent development of complications, such as gross atelectasis, pneumonia and respiratory failure. Studies have indicated that these conditions can be reversed by hyperinflation of the lungs through deep breathing with a prolonged inspiratory phase.

Indications for Lung Expansion

Patients who are most likely to benefit from lung expansion assistance are those who are unable or unwilling to take a deep breath because of pain, sedation or neuromuscular disorders. Patients with chronically decreased lung compliance due to conditions, such as obesity, chest wall deformity or fibrotic lung disease, are also frequently assisted with lung expansion maneuvers. A major group of patients who tend to breathe at a low, constant tidal volume because of pain and/or sedation are those who have undergone thoracic and abdominal surgery. In most hospitals, such patients are routinely administered either IPPB or incentive spirometry.

For many years, the primary method of assisting surgical and medical patients with lung expansion was by means of IPPB. More recently, however, many hospitals are replacing IPPB with incentive spirometry except for patients who are unable or unwilling to achieve lung expansion without medical assistance. This replacement has occurred because incentive spirometry is simpler and less expensive to administer and because much controversy exists over the efficacy of IPPB as a therapeutic modality.

Regardless of the method used, further research is needed to establish the effectiveness of lung expansion therapy in general. Whatever benefits patients receive from either IPPB or incentive spirometry may be indirect in nature. The apparent benefits may result from such factors as clearance of secretions, repositioning of the body or the psychological effects of interaction with the therapist. Although the benefits of lung expansion assistance may not be solely physiological in nature, the therapy may still be worthwhile because of the patient's feeling of improvement.

In this module, we have focused our attention on only two methods of lung expansion assistance. The use of blow bottles, CPAP and PEEP were intentionally omitted from this module. Blow bottle therapy was left out because there is no convincing evidence that this procedure accomplishes hyperinflation. The physiological rationale for CPAP appears sound, but the procedure is used primarily for infants at the present time and is included in **Module 15.0**. Since PEEP is an adjunct to ventilator care, it is included with continuous mechanical ventilation in **Module 13.0.**

Clinical Procedure 11.1
Incentive Spirometry

An incentive spirometer is a device used to encourage and monitor the performance of deep, sustained, voluntary inspirations. Since inspiration is voluntary, the same effects can be accomplished without an incentive spirometer. The device is useful, however, because it enables the patient to see the volume of air inspired. The purpose of this visual evidence is to provide motivation for patient cooperation. Incentive spirometry has been found especially useful in motivating patients who have difficulty taking deep breaths because of such factors as pain and fatigue.

Let's consider the factors which tend to influence the effectiveness of incentive spirometry. First, a sufficient volume of air should be inspired to inflate the alveoli as completely as possible. This volume will vary with the size and conditions of the patient but, ordinarily, it should be at least twice the patient's normal tidal volume. It is also believed that the effectiveness of incentive spirometry is enhanced by pausing at end-inspiration to sustain hyperinflation. For these reasons, incentive spirometers are designed to encourage the patient to take as deep a breath as possible and to hold it for at least two to three seconds.

Procedure for Performing Incentive Spirometry

The following procedure is recommended for use whenever incentive spirometry is prescribed for a patient:

A. *Check Order.* Verify the physician's order as follows:

1. Compare the requisition with the physician's order to ensure that no discrepancies exist.

2. Review the order to ensure that the following are prescribed:

   • Tidal volume
   • Frequency of therapy
   • Duration of therapy

3. If any part of the order is unfamiliar, question its accuracy.

B. **Review Chart.** Use the following procedure to review the patient's chart:

1. On the patient's chart, identify all pertinent data in the following areas:

   • History and physical
   • Admitting diagnosis
   • Progress notes
   • Blood gas analysis
   • Chest x-rays

C. **Maintain Asepsis.** While performing the remainder of this procedure, you are expected to maintain aseptic conditions and follow universal precautions according to the procedure described in **SSE 1.2.** This includes washing your hands:

• Before obtaining equipment
• Following performance of **K. Conclude Procedure**
• Anytime during the procedure that contamination is suspected

D. **Obtain Equipment.** Collect the following equipment and supplies:

• Incentive spirometer
• Mouthpiece
• Mainstream tubing
• Stethoscope

E. **Assemble Equipment.** Prepare the equipment for use as follows:

1. Connect the mainstream tubing between:

   • Mouthpiece
   • Spirometer outlet

F. **Test Equipment.** Test the incentive spirometry equipment as follows:

1. Depending on the equipment used, perform the appropriate test as follows:

   • Flush the bell to assure that it moves freely
   • Check the lights and fuses on the digital spirometer
   • Make certain all moving parts are functional

G. ***Confirm Patient.*** Ensure that the procedure is performed with the correct patient as follows:

1. Match the information on the order with the following:

   • Room number
   • Name on the door or bed
   • Name on the wristband

2. Greet the patient by name (in a questioning manner if unknown).

3. Resolve any discrepancies in the patient identification information by conferring with the nursing staff.

H. ***Inform Patient.*** Interact with the patient as follows:

1. Introduce yourself by name and department (if not already acquainted).

2. Tell the patient what procedure is to be performed.

3. Explain the procedure by describing:

   • What is to be performed
   • How it will be performed
   • What the patient is expected to do
   • What you will be doing
   • How frequently it will be performed

I. ***Implement Procedure.*** Perform the following tasks:

1. Position the patient in an upright position (45 to 90° angle).

2. Coach the patient to breathe in the following manner:

   • Diaphragmatically
   • Through the mouth
   • Slowly and deeply
   • Pause at end-inspiration, maintaining an I:E ratio of at least 1:2

J. ***Monitor Patient.*** Determine the patient's response to the therapy as follows:

1. Determine the pulse rate. (Count for at least one minute.)

2. Determine the respiratory rate. (Count for at least one minute.)

3. Auscultate the patient's chest according to the procedure described in **SSE 2.2**.

4. Note any abnormalities in the patient's appearance or behavior.

K. *Conclude Procedure.* Complete the following tasks:

1. Place the patient in a comfortable position.

2. Assure that the call bell and bedside table are within the patient's reach.

3. Ask if the patient has any needs.

4. Answer any questions as effectively as possible.

5. Unplug and cover the equipment and move it away from the patient's bed (or remove it from the room).

L. *Record Results.* Document the therapy as follows:

1. Record the following data on the patient's chart:

   • Date
   • Time
   • Therapy administered
   • Pulse rate
   • Respiratory rate
   • Abnormal patient characteristics
   • Therapy-related patient complaints

2. Sign the patient's chart (first initial and full last name).

M. *Report Observations.* Report the following information:

1. Report any significant adverse changes in the patient's conditions to the nurse or physician whenever observed.

2. Following the procedure, inform the appropriate personnel of:

   • Patient requests
   • Patient complaints
   • Unexpressed patient needs

3. Following the procedure, report to the nurse or physician:

   • Any non-critical adverse reactions to the therapy
   • Other pertinent observations of the patient's condition

Clinical Procedure 11.2
Intermittent Positive Pressure Breathing

Intermittent positive pressure breathing (IPPB) refers to the use of a ventilator to enhance lung expansion during inspiration. The inspiratory effort of a patient causes the ventilator to deliver pressurized room air or supplemental oxygen. The gas is delivered until a predetermined pressure in the patient's airway is reached. At that time, the ventilator cycles off, allowing the patient to exhale passively.

The effectiveness of IPPB therapy appears to be influenced by at least three factors: (1) the volume of air delivered, (2) the timing of expiration, and (3) the frequency of administration. Because IPPB machines are pressure-cycled, it is necessary to monitor the volume of air delivered in order to ensure adequate lung expansion. It may also be necessary to instruct the patient in breath-holding techniques in order to sustain a state of hyperinflation. In addition, it has been suggested that IPPB be administered at least hourly for maximally beneficial effects. Failure to address any of these factors may be responsible for the belief that IPPB therapy has limited effectiveness.

One of the early uses of IPPB was in the treatment of patients with chronic obstructive pulmonary disease (COPD). Because many COPD patients have increased lung compliance and a loss of airway elasticity, the physiological rationale for using IPPB for such patients is quite different from the rationale for administering IPPB therapy to post-surgical and other medical patients. Due to the cost of administering IPPB and its questionable efficacy for COPD patients, except as a means of delivering medications, its use for this purpose has declined dramatically during the last few years.

Hazards and Precautions

The most common side effect of IPPB therapy is hyperventilation. When breathing an increased volume, a significant decrease in the respiratory rate is necessary in order to reduce the incidence of hyperventilation. In addition, there is always the possibility of pneumothorax or complications resulting from gastric distention during the application of positive airway pressure. Most of the other hazards related to IPPB therapy are attributable to the medications delivered (see **CPE 10.3**) or the use of supplemental oxygen (see **CPE 9.1**). Whenever any of these adverse responses are observed during the administration of IPPB therapy, the procedure should be stopped immediately and the physician notified.

Procedure for Performing IPPB Therapy

The following procedure is recommended for performing IPPB therapy whenever it is prescribed for a patient:

A. ***Check Order.*** Verify the physician's order as follows:

   1. Compare the requisition with the physician's order to ensure that no discrepancies exist.

   2. Review the order to ensure that the following are prescribed:

      * Frequency of therapy
      * Medication and dosage
      * Tidal volume of inspiratory pressure

   3. If any part of the order is unfamiliar, question its accuracy.

B. ***Review Chart.*** Use the following procedure to review the patient's chart:

   1. On the patient's chart, identify all pertinent data in the following areas:

      * History and physical
      * Admitting diagnosis
      * Progress notes
      * Blood gas analysis
      * Chest x-rays

   2. Based on the patient data, identify the following:

      * Conditions that indicate the need for IPPB therapy
      * Potential hazards of IPPB therapy for the patient

C. ***Maintain Asepsis.*** While performing the remainder of this procedure, you are expected to maintain aseptic conditions and follow universal precautions according to the procedure described in **SSE 1.2**. This includes washing your hands:

   * Before obtaining equipment
   * Following performance of ***K. Conclude Procedure***
   * Anytime during the procedure that contamination is suspected

D. **Obtain Equipment.** Collect the following equipment and supplies:

- Ventilator
- Mainstream tubing
- Nebulizer and exhalation valve tubing
- Manifold and nebulizer
- Patient attachment and flex tube
- Test lung
- Medication
- Volume measuring device with appropriate adaptor
- High pressure hose and gas source connectors
- Stethoscope

Note: *The next two steps (E and F) will vary according to the type of equipment ordered. Proceed with the set of steps which corresponds with the equipment prescribed for the patient.*

BIRD RESPIRATORS

E. **Assemble Equipment.** Prepare the equipment for use as follows:

1. Connect the mainstream tubing to the mainstream outlet.

2. Attach the other end of the mainstream tubing to the patient manifold.

3. Connect the nebulizer power drive line to the nebulizer outlet.

4. Attach the other end of the nebulizer power drive line to the nebulizer tee.

5. Attach the high pressure tubing to the gas inlet on the ventilator.

6. Attach the test lung to the patient manifold.

F. **Test Equipment.** Test the **Bird** equipment as follows:

1. Turn all controls off.

2. Plug the high pressure tubing into the correct gas source.

3. Set the system pressure above 10 cm H_2O.

4. Adjust the inspiratory flow knob by turning it 180°.

5. Adjust the sensitivity so that a slight squeeze of the test lung will cycle the respirator into the inspiratory phase.

6. If the ventilator does not cycle off when manually cycled, increase the flow rate and repeat.

7. If the ventilator still does not cycle off, tighten all connections and repeat.

8. If the ventilator still does not cycle off, change circuits and repeat.

9. If the ventilator still does not cycle off:

    a. Label the ventilator as "defective" and replace it.
    b. Reassemble and retest the new equipment.

10. Remove the test lung and instill the prescribed medication into the nebulizer.

11. Manually cycle the ventilator by pushing in the hand timer rod.

12. If a fine mist does not appear, change nebulizer and repeat.

BENNETT RESPIRATORS

E. *Assemble Equipment.* Prepare the equipment for use as follows:

1. Connect the mainstream tubing to the mainstream outlet.

2. Attach the other end of the mainstream tubing to the patient manifold.

3. Connect the nebulizer tubing to the nebulizer outlet.

4. Attach the other end of the nebulizer tubing to the nebulizer.

5. Connect the exhalation valve tubing to the exhalation valve outlet.

6. Attach the other end of the exhalation valve tubing to the exhalation valve.

7. Attach the high pressure tubing to the gas inlet on the ventilator.

F. *Test Equipment.* Test the **Bennett** IPPB equipment as follows:

1. Turn all controls off.

2. Plug the high pressure tubing into the correct gas source.

3. Set the system pressure above 10 cm H_2O.

4. Manually cycle the ventilator by slightly squeezing the test lung to create a subambient pressure.

5. If the ventilator does not cycle off, tighten all connections.

6. If the ventilator still does not cycle off and the **Bennett** valve moves freely, change circuits and repeat.

7. If the ventilator still does not cycle off and the **Bennett** valve does not move freely, clean the valve.

8. If the ventilator still does not cycle off after changing circuits and cleaning the valve:

   a. Label the ventilator as "defective" and replace it.
   b. Reassemble and retest the new equipment.

9. Remove the test lung and instill the prescribed medication into the nebulizer.

10. Turn on the nebulizer.

11. If the fine mist is absent, change the nebulizer and repeat.

Note: *Using the ventilator that you have assembled and tested, complete the IPPB treatment according to the following procedures.*

G. **Confirm Patient.** Ensure that the procedure is performed on the correct patient as follows:

1. Match the information on the order with the following:

   • Room number
   • Name on the door or bed
   • Name on the wristband

2. Greet the patient by name (in a questioning manner if unknown).

3. Resolve any discrepancies in the patient identification information by conferring with the nursing staff.

H. **Inform Patient.** Interact with the patient as follows:

1. Introduce yourself by name and department (if not already acquainted).

2. Tell the patient what procedure is to be performed.

3. Explain the procedure by describing:

- Why it is to be performed
- How it will be performed
- What the patient is expected to do
- What you will be doing
- How frequently it will be performed

I. **_Implement Procedure._** Perform the following tasks:

1. Position the patient in an upright position (45 to 90° angle).

2. Administer IPPB therapy as follows:

   a. Plug the high pressure tubing into the correct gas source.
   b. Adjust the inspiratory pressure control to the prescribed pressure.
   c. Attach the IPPB therapy device to the patient.

3. Coach the patient to breathe in the following manner:

   - Diaphragmatically
   - Slowly and deeply
   - Allow the machine to cycle off before initiating expiration
   - Pause at end-inspiration, maintaining an I:E ratio of at least 1:2

J. **_Monitor Patient._** Determine the patient's response to the therapy as follows:

1. Determine the pulse rate. (Count for at least one minute.)

2. Determine the respiratory rate. (Count for at least one minute.)

3. Observe respirations to identify any abnormalities in the breathing pattern.

4. Measure the patient's exhaled tidal volume. Adjust the system pressure to obtain a tidal volume of 8 to 15 cc/kg body weight.

5. Auscultate the patient's chest according to the procedure described in **SSE 2.2.**

6. Note any abnormalities in the patient's appearance or behavior.

K. *Conclude Procedure.* Complete the following tasks:

1. Place the patient in a comfortable position.

2. Assure that the call bell and bedside table are within the patient's reach.

3. Ask if the patient has any needs.

4. Answer any questions as effectively as possible.

5. Unplug and cover the equipment and move it away from the patient's bedside (or remove it from the room).

L. *Record Results.* Document the therapy as follows:

1. Record the following data on the patient's chart:

   - Date
   - Time
   - Therapy administered
   - Inspiratory pressure
   - Tidal volume
   - FIO_2
   - Pulse rate
   - Respiratory rate
   - Abnormal patient characteristics
   - Therapy-related patient complaints
   - Volume, color and consistency of sputum produced

2. Sign the patient's chart (first initial and full last name).

M. *Report Observations.* Report the following information:

1. Report any significant adverse changes in the patient's condition to the nurse or physician whenever observed.

2. Following the procedure, inform the appropriate personnel of:

   - Patient requests
   - Patient complaints
   - Unexpressed patient needs

3. Following the procedure, report to the nurse or physician:

   - Any non-critical adverse reactions to the therapy
   - Other pertinent observations of the patient's condition

Evaluation of Lung Expansion Therapy Procedures

The following definitions are provided for use whenever the respective Lung Expansion Therapy Procedures are evaluated. In order for performance of the procedures to be considered acceptable, all Essential Tasks must be performed according to the accompanying Evaluation Criteria. Any deviation from the following task sequence or criteria must be approved by the evaluator.

CPE 11.1 Incentive Spirometry		
Performance	**Essential Tasks**	**Evaluation Criteria**
A. Check Order	See **SSE 3.1**	See **SSE 3.1**
B. Review Chart	See **SSE 3.2**	See **SSE 3.2**
C. Maintain Asepsis	See **SSE 1.2**	See **SSE 1.2**
D. Obtain Equipment	1. Obtains the following equipment and supplies: • Incentive spirometer • Mouthpiece • Mainstream tubing • Stethoscope	a. Correct equipment obtained
E. Assemble Equipment	1. Connects tubing to: • Mouthpiece • Spirometer outlet	a. Assembled according to order and **SOP**
F. Test Equipment	1. Tests for: • Free movement • Functioning of lights and fuses • Functioning of moving patients	a. Tested according to **SOP**
G. Confirm Patient	See **SSE 3.3**	See **SSE 3.3**

CPE 11.1
Incentive Spirometry (continued)

Performance	Essential Tasks	Evaluation Criteria
H. Inform Patient	See SSE 4.1	See SSE 4.1
I. Implement Procedure	1. Positions patient	a. Placed in upright position (45-90°)
	2. Coaches patient to breathe: • Diaphragmatically • Through the mouth • Slowly and deeply • Pause at end-inspiration	a. Clear and accurate instructions provided b. Patient performance encouraged c. Instructions repeated as needed
J. Monitor Patient	1. Determines: • Pulse rate • Respiratory rate	a. Counted for at least one (1) minute.
	2. Auscultates chest	a. Performed according to SSE 2.2
	3. Observes patient appearance	a. Any abnormalities identified
K. Conclude Procedure	1. Restores room to original condition	a. Equipment removed from room or covered and moved to suitable location within room b. Call bell and bedside table positioned within patient's reach
	2. Tends to patient needs	a. Comfortable position assured b. Patient asked regarding other needs c. Patient questions answered effectively
L. Record Results	See SSE 3.4	See SSE 3.4
M. Report Observations	See SSE 4.3	See SSE 4.3

CPE 11.2
Intermittent Positive Pressure Breathing

Performance	Essential Tasks	Evaluation Criteria
A. Check Order	See SSE 3.1	See SSE 3.1
B. Review Chart	See SSE 3.2	See SSE 3.2
C. Maintain Asepsis	See SSE 1.2	See SSE 1.2
D. Obtain Equipment	1. Obtains the following equipment and supplies: • Ventilator • Mainstream tubing • Nebulizer and exhalation valve tubing • Patient attachment and flex valve tubing • Test lung • Medication • Volume measuring device • High pressure hose and connector • Stethoscope	a. Correct equipment obtained
E. Assemble Equipment	1. Prepares equipment as follows: • Attaches IPPB circuit to ventilator • Attaches test lung to manifold	a. Assembled according to order and **SOP**
F. Test Equipment	1. Tests for: • Leaks in system • Functioning of valve (**Bennett**) • Functioning of nebulizer	a. Tested according to **SOP** b. Leaks remedied c. Fine mist produced d. Defective equipment replaced
G. Confirm Patient	See SSE 3.3	See SSE 3.3

CPE 11.2 Intermitent Positive Pressure Breathing (continued)		
Performance	**Essential Tasks**	**Evaluation Criteria**
H. Inform Patient	See SSE 4.1	See SSE 4.1
I. Implement Procedure	1. Positions patient	a. Placed in upright position (45-90°)
	2. Administers therapy	a. Correct pressure used b. Delivery device attached correctly
	3. Coaches patient to breathe: • Diaphragmatically • Through the mouth • Slowly and deeply • Pause at end-inspiration	a. Clear and accurate instructions provided b. Patient performance encouraged c. Instructions repeated as needed
J. Monitor Patient	1. Determines: • Pulse rate • Respiratory rate.	a. Counted for at least one (1) minute b. Repeated at 5-10 minute intervals
	2. Observes: • Respiratory pattern • Patient appearance	a. Any abnormalities identified
	3. Measures exhaled tidal volume	a. Tidal volume measured tidal volume accurately b. Tidal volume of 8-15 ml\kg body weight obtained
K. Conclude Procedure	1. Restores room to original condition	a. Equipment removed from room or covered and moved to suitable location within room b. Call bell and bedside table positioned within patient's reach
	2. Tends to patient needs	a. Comfortable position assured b. Patient asked regarding other needs c. Patient questions answered effectively
L. Record Results	See SSE 3.4	See SSE 3.4
M. Report Observations	See SSE 4.3	See SSE 4.3

Module 12.0

Chest Physical Therapy

Retention of tracheobronchial secretions is a major problem of patients with pulmonary disorders. The presence of these retained secretions reduces ventilatory efficiency by obstructing airways thereby restricting air flow and reducing gas exchange. Postural drainage, chest percussion, and coughing facilitate the mobilization and removal of bronchial secretions. The purpose of this module is to assure proficiency in performing these basic chest physical therapy procedures.

Objectives

Upon completion of this module, you will be able to:

1. Describe the importance of bronchial hygiene.

2. List the indications and hazards of chest percussion and postural drainage.

3. Perform chest percussion and postural drainage procedures as prescribed for a patient.

One commonly performed physical therapy procedure is postural drainage with percussion. This procedure is used with surgical and acutely ill medical patients, as well as patients with chronic pulmonary disorders. Patients who receive this therapy are all characterized by the presence of excessive quantities of tracheobronchial secretions.

The normal human body continuously produces tracheobronchial secretions at a rate of approximately 100 ml per day. These mucoidal secretions provide an essential protective covering of the tracheobronchial epithelium. Ordinarily, these secretions are mobilized by the constant escalatory action of the ciliated lining of the airway. There are times, however, when the secretions tend to build up in the airway because they are produced in excessive amounts due to bronchopulmonary disorders. At other times, excessive tenacity of the secretions or ineffective removal mechanisms may result in a build up. In any of these circumstances, chest physical therapy can be highly beneficial.

Clinical Procedure 12.1
Chest Percussion
and Postural Drainage

Before describing chest physical therapy procedures, we should first discuss the natural defense mechanism against retained secretions, the cough. When performed with sufficient force, this natural mechanism is the most effective method of clearing secretions from the airway. The cough is normally stimulated by tracheal or bronchial irritation resulting from secretions retained in the airway. Although coughing is a natural response, many patients can be taught to improve the effectiveness of the cough mechanism.

Secretions that are loosened and mobilized during chest physical therapy procedures must be evacuated from the airway. Although tracheal suctioning may sometimes be required to remove these secretions, they can usually be expelled by the cough mechanism. When administering chest physical therapy, the patient should be encouraged to expectorate, not swallow, the sputum. The amount, color, and consistency of the sputum should be noted.

Postural Drainage

Much of the movement of secretions by the cilia is in a direction opposite the force of gravity. By properly positioning the body, the force of gravity can be used to enhance, rather than impede, the movement of secretions. This procedure of placing the body in a posture that facilitates the flow of secretions into the larger airways where they can be more easily expectorated is called postural drainage. Because the direction of secretion movement varies throughout the generations of bronchi, several different positions are needed to facilitate drainage of different segments of the lungs. These positions are discussed in detail in the evaluation portion of this module.

Indications

The general conditions that indicate the need for postural drainage include the following:

1. Excessive production of bronchial secretions due to conditions such as cystic fibrosis, bronchiectasis, or pneumonia.

2. Inability to expel tracheobronchial secretions adequately because of an ineffective cough mechanism resulting from conditions such as neurological impairment, muscular weakness or emphysema.

Contraindications and Hazards

For some patients, there are risks associated with the movement of certain parts of the body or with the assuming of certain body positions. Therefore, the potential benefits of postural drainage must outweigh the potential risks when applying this technique. Postural drainage cannot be considered for patients with conditions requiring total immobilization of the body. For other patients, certain postural drainage positions may be contraindicated. Still other patients may be candidates for postural drainage, but certain predisposing conditions can create situations that are potentially hazardous for the patient. Postural drainage should be avoided or used with caution under the following circumstances:

Contraindications: The contraindications for postural drainage are:

1. The presence of conditions requiring total immobilization such as spinal, cranial, or ophthalmic surgery or injury.

2. The presence of conditions which prevent the patient from assuming certain postural drainage positions. These include pulmonary edema, orthopedic conditions requiring traction or partial immobilization, and conditions which may be adversely affected by increased intracranial pressure.

Hazards: The following potential hazards of postural drainage should be considered:

1. Increased work of breathing due to positional restriction of the respiratory muscles.

2. Partial airway obstruction due to rapid and extensive accumulation of mobilized secretions.

3. Physiological stress to the cardiovascular system in patients with pre-existing cardiac or circulatory abnormalities.

There are times when the therapeutic value of postural drainage may be outweighed by adverse patient reactions to the procedure. Some patients may experience dyspnea, pain, or anxiety when placed in certain positions. These conditions can often be avoided or reduced by providing the patient with careful handling and assurance. If the conditions persist, the procedure should be discontinued.

Chest Percussion

In most instances, postural drainage alone will not adequately mobilize tracheobronchial secretions. Due to the consistency and tenacity of retained secretions, it may be necessary to employ a concomitant procedure to loosen them. The technique most commonly used in conjunction with postural drainage is chest percussion. This technique involves the generation of sound waves by rhythmically striking the chest wall with cupped hands. Air vibrations are transmitted throughout the thoracic cavity to loosen adherent secretions.

Chest percussion is performed by rapidly striking the chest wall with cupped hands. When properly performed, the procedure produces a hollow popping sound with a regular rhythm. Although chest percussion should not be painful, it is sometimes desirable to cushion the blows by covering the chest wall with a towel or similar protective material. Care should be taken to keep the patient comfortable and to avoid percussing areas susceptible to injury. These areas include the spinal column, sternum, clavicles, scapula, kidneys, abdomen, floating ribs, and female breast tissue.

Indications

The conditions that indicate the need for chest percussion include the following:

1. The presence of thick and tenacious tracheobronchial secretions produced by conditions such as bronchiectasis, lung abscess, chronic bronchitis, or cystic fibrosis.

2. The inability to loosen tracheobronchial secretions because of an ineffective cough mechanism resulting from such factors as emphysema, neurological impairment, or muscular weakness.

Contraindications and Hazards

Although chest percussion appears to be useful for loosening adherent secretions, it cannot be used indiscriminately with all patients. As in the case of postural drainage, certain conditions contraindicate the use of chest percussion and other conditions necessitate proceeding with caution. Chest percussion should be avoided or used with caution under the following circumstances:

Contraindications: The contraindications for chest percussion are:

1. The presence of severe osteoporosis resulting from such factors as estrogen deficiency or long-term steroid therapy.

2. The presence of lung tissue conditions such as hemoptysis or resectable tumors.

3. The presence of untreated pleural disorders such as pneumothorax or extensive empyema.

Hazards: The potential hazards of chest percussion are:

1. Injury to internal organs as a result of percussing beyond the thoracic cavity.

2. Injury to bones and connective tissue surrounding the thoracic cavity due to over-vigorous percussion or extremely fragile body structures.

3. Disturbance of dressings, sutures, and drainage tubes associated with thoracic surgery or trauma.

4. Inducing unnecessary pain when percussing areas made sensitive by such factors as trauma or disease.

Even when performed correctly and with due caution, chest percussion procedures can cause minor discomfort and produce anxiety for apprehensive patients. As with postural drainage, these conditions can often be avoided or reduced by careful handling of the patient. If the patient experiences excessive discomfort or anxiety, the procedure should be discontinued and the physician notified.

Other Procedures

Chest physical therapy includes other techniques designed to improve breathing efficiency. These techniques are seldom prescribed as separate procedures but are usually performed whenever the need arises during the administration of other therapy. For this reason, methods of training patients to improve their breathing efficiency are presented as Ancillary Procedures.

During the removal of retained secretions, it is sometimes necessary to employ tracheal suctioning procedures. Suctioning is a routinely performed airway management procedure and is not considered a form of chest physical therapy.

Procedure for Performing Chest Percussion and Postural Drainage

Chest physical therapy in the form of postural drainage accompanied by chest percussion is performed as follows:

A. *Check Order.* Verify the physician's order as follows:

    1. Compare the requisition with the physician's order to ensure that no discrepancies exist.

    2. Review the order to ensure that the following are prescribed:

        • Frequency of therapy
        • Areas of the lungs to be percussed and drained

    3. If any part of the order is unfamiliar, question its accuracy.

B. *Review Chart.* Use the following procedure to review the patient's chart:

    1. On the patient's chart, identify all pertinent data in the following areas:

        • History and physical
        • Admitting diagnosis
        • Progress notes
        • Blood gas analysis

    2. Based on the patient data, identify the following:

        • Conditions that indicate the need for chest physical therapy
        • Potential hazards of chest physical therapy for the patient

C. *Maintain Asepsis.* While performing the remainder of this procedure, you are expected to maintain aseptic conditions and follow universal precautions according to the procedure described in **SSE 1.2.** This includes washing your hands:

    • Before obtaining equipment
    • Following performance of step *I. Conclude Procedure*
    • Anytime during the procedure that contamination is suspected

D. **_Obtain Equipment._** Collect the following equipment and supplies:

- Towel or similar protective material
- Stethoscope

E. **_Confirm Patient._** Ensure that the procedure is performed on the correct patient as follows:

1. Match the information on the order with the following:

   - Room number
   - Name on the door or bed
   - Name on the wristband

2. Greet the patient by name (in a questioning manner if unknown).

3. Resolve any discrepancies in the patient identification information by conferring with the nursing staff.

Table 12-1
Lung Segments and Accompanying Positions
for Percussion and Drainage

Position	Lung	Lobe	Segment	Body Position
1	Right	Upper	Apical	Sitting
	Left	Upper		Leaning back 30°
2	Right	Upper	Posterior	Sitting
	Left	Upper		Leaning back 30°
3	Right	Upper	Anterior	Supine
	Left	Upper		Pillow under knees
4	Right	Lower	Superior	Prone
5	Right	Middle	Lateral	With foot of bed elevated 15°: Right oblique (rotate patient as necessary)
			Medial	
6	Left		Lingula	With foot of bed elevated 15°: Left oblique (rotate patient as necessary)
7	Right	Lower	Lateral basal	With foot of bed elevated 15°:
	Left	Lower	Posterior basal	Right oblique
			Anterior basal	Left oblique

F.   *Inform Patient.* Interact with the patient as follows:

    1. Introduce yourself by name and department (if not already acquainted).

    2. Tell the patient what procedure is to be performed.

    3. Explain the procedure by describing:

        • Why it is to be performed
        • How it will be performed
        • What the patient is expected to do
        • What you will be doing
        • How frequently it will be performed

G.   *Implement Procedure.* Perform the following tasks:

1. Auscultate the chest according to the procedure described in **SSE 2.2**.

2. Select the lung segment to be percussed and drained by following the position sequence given in ***Table 12-1***.

3. Position the patient as indicated in ***Table 12-1*** for the lung segment to be percussed by providing instructions and assistance.

4. Move your hands along the patient's chest wall to define the lung segment boundaries.

5. With cupped hands, percuss over the defined lung segment, avoiding areas susceptible to injury.

6. Encourage the patient to cough following percussion of each lung segment.

7. Repeat Steps 2 through 6 until all lung segments requiring therapy have been percussed and drained.

H.   *Monitor Patient.* Determine the patient's response to the therapy as follows:

    1. Determine the pulse rate. (Count for at least one minute).

    2. Determine the respiratory rate. (Count for at least one minute).

    3. Observe respirations to identify any abnormalities in the breathing pattern.

4. Auscultate the chest according to the procedure described in **SSE 2.2**. Repeat percussion over any areas where adventitious breath sounds are audible.

5. Note any abnormalities in the patient's appearance or behavior.

I. Conclude Procedure. Complete the following tasks:

1. Place the patient in a comfortable position.

2. Assure that the call bell and bedside table are within the patient's reach.

3. Ask if the patient has any needs.

4. Answer any questions as effectively as possible.

J. Record Results. Document the therapy as follows:

1. Record the following data on the patient's chart:

   • Date
   • Time
   • Therapy administered
   • Pulse rate
   • Respiratory rate
   • Volume, color, and consistency of sputum
   • Abnormal patient characteristics
   • Therapy-related patient complaints

2. Sign the patient's chart (first initial and full last name).

K. Report Observations. Report the following information:

1. Report any significant adverse changes in the patient's condition to the nurse or physician whenever observed.

2. Following the procedure, inform the appropriate personnel of:

   • Patient requests
   • Patient complaints
   • Unexpressed patient needs

3. Following the procedure, report to the nurse or physician:

   • Any non-critical adverse reactions to the therapy
   • Other pertinent observations of the patient's condition

Evaluation of Chest Physical Therapy Procedures

The following definitions are provided for use whenever the respective Chest Physical Therapy Procedures are evaluated. In order for performance of the procedures to be considered acceptable, all Essential Tasks must be performed according to the accompanying Evaluation Criteria. Any deviation from the following task sequence or criteria must be approved by the evaluator.

CPE 12.1 Chest Percussion and Postural Drainage		
Performance	**Essential Tasks**	**Evaluation Criteria**
A. Check Order	See SSE 3.1	See SSE 3.1
B. Review Chart	See SSE 3.2	See SSE 3.2
C. Maintain Asepsis	See SSE 1.2	See SSE 1.2
D. Obtain Equipment	1. Obtains the following equipment and supplies: • Towel • Stethoscope	a. Correct equipment obtained
E. Confirm Patient	See SSE 3.3	See SSE 3.3
F. Inform Patient	See SSE 4.1	See SSE 4.1
G. Implement Procedure	1. Auscultates chest	a. Performed according to SSE 2.2
	2. Selects lung segments	a. Correct sequence followed (**Table 12.1**)
	3. Positions patient	a. Positioned correctly for lung segment (**Table 12.1**)

CPE 12.1
Chest Percussion and Postural Drainage (continued)

Performance	Essential Tasks	Evaluation Criteria
G. Implement Procedure (continued)	4. Defines lung boundaries	a. Boundaries correctly defined for lung segment
	5. Percusses defined lung segment	a. Hands cupped correctly b. Acceptable rate and rhythm of percussion used c. Appropriate striking force applied d. Performed within lung boundaries e. Injury-prone areas avoided
	6. Encourages coughing following percussion of each segment	a. Clear and complete instructions provided b. Instructions repeated when necessary
	7. Repeats procedure	a. All lung segments percussed and drained b. Performed in correct sequence c. All steps performed correctly
H. Monitor Patient	1. Determines: • Pulse rate • Respiratory rate	a. Counted for at least one (1) minute
	2. Observes: • Respiratory pattern • Patient appearance	a. Any abnormalities identified
	3. Auscultates chest	a. Performed according to SSE 2.2 b. Repeats percussion over any areas where adventitious sounds are audible
I. Conclude Procedure	1. Replaces call bell and bedside table	a. Placed within patient's reach
	2. Tends to patient needs	a. Comfortable position assured b. Patient asked regarding other needs c. Patient questions answered effectively

CPE 12.1		
Chest Percussion and Postural Drainage (continued)		
Performance	Essential Tasks	Evaluation Criteria
J. Record Results	See SSE 3.4	See SSE 3.4
K. Report Observations	See SSE 4.3	See SSE 4.3

Module 13.0

Ventilator Management

Continuous mechanical ventilation is used to control or assist the respiration of patients who are unable to maintain an adequate ventilatory status because of some underlying disease or physical condition. The procedure reduces the work of breathing and improves ventilatory efficiency by manipulating the respiratory pattern and airway pressures. Respiratory care personnel must be able to perform all tasks associated with providing ventilatory support for a patient. The purpose of this module is to ensure your proficiency in the preparation and use of a mechanical ventilator for providing continuous ventilation with or without the use of positive end-expiratory pressure (PEEP) or intermittent mandatory ventilation (IMV).

Objectives

Upon completion of this module, you will be able to:

1. List the indications and hazards of continuous mechanical ventilation, IMV and PEEP.

2. Perform the tasks required to set up a ventilator for patient use.

3. Perform the equipment and patient monitoring procedures required to ensure proper ventilator functioning and to evaluate patient status and response to therapy.

4. Perform a routine change-out of a ventilator circuit.

5. Provide positive end-expiratory pressure to a patient receiving continuous mechanical ventilation.

6. Provide intermittent mandatory ventilation to a ventilator patient.

Life-sustaining metabolic processes involve many oxidative chemical reactions in which oxygen is consumed and carbon dioxide is produced. In order for these reactions to occur, oxygen must be removed from the atmosphere, diffused into the blood stream and transported to the sites where the reactions take place. Simultaneously, the carbon dioxide produced by the reactions must be transported to the lungs, diffused into the alveoli and released into the atmosphere. For this gas exchange to occur, air must continuously enter and exit the lungs by the process of ventilation.

Atmospheric gases flow into and out of the lungs as a result of pressure changes in the thoracic cavity. When the cavity is expanded by the contraction of the respiratory muscles, the pressure is decreased causing air to flow into the lungs. The gases are expelled as the muscles relax, allowing the cavity to return to its resting shape and size. Failure of the body to correctly perform any of these steps may necessitate ventilatory assistance.

The most obvious and most critical condition requiring ventilatory support is apnea. Other less-severe patient conditions may also necessitate providing mechanical assistance with breathing. For example limitations, either in the functioning of the respiratory muscles or in the ability of the lungs or chest wall to expand, will restrict the volume of air entering the lungs during inspiration. In this situation, a mechanical ventilator can be used to force air or supplemental oxygen into the lungs. In other situations, mechanical ventilation may be necessary to reverse the conditions leading to acute respiratory failure. By increasing the rate or depth of an individual's respiratory pattern, a ventilator can assist in removing excess carbon dioxide from the lungs.

The Nature of Ventilatory Assistance

Mechanical ventilators are designed to provide a patient with varying degrees of ventilatory assistance. The degree of assistance ranges from adjusting the triggering sensitivity to enable the patient to initiate each breath to totally controlling respiration. In the former situation, the respiratory rate of the ventilator is set slightly below the patient's rate to assure continuity of respiration in case the patient's rate should decrease. Total control of respiration is necessary when the patient is apneic or when the chest wall needs to be stabilized, as in the case of a severe flail chest.

In general, continuous mechanical ventilation attempts to simulate the normal breathing pattern of an individual. This includes the regulation of respiratory rate, flow rate and I:E ratio. Ordinarily, the respiratory rate is ordered by the physician. Respiratory care personnel will then adjust the flow rate in order to establish an appropriate I:E ratio. In making this adjustment, it should be remembered that increasing the flow rate in an effort to decrease inspiratory time also tends to increase turbulent flow. Except for patients with extremely low pulmonary compliance, therefore, the flow rate should be adjusted as low as possible while still maintaining an acceptable I:E ratio.

Mechanical Ventilation Equipment

Thereare two major types of mechanical ventilators in use today, pressure-limited and volume-limited. Both machines assist the patient with with inspiration by delivering air or supplemental oxygen with positive pressure. They differ in the method by which the inspiratory phase of the breathing cycle is terminated. A pressure-limited ventilator delivers gas until a predetermined pressure is reached, while a volume-limited ventilator delivers a predetermined volume of gas regardless of the pressure generated.

The volume of gas delivered by a pressure-limited ventilator varies with the patient's pulmonary compliance. Because of this characteristic, the ventilation provided by such a machine tends to be inconsistent. To ensure the delivery of a constant, adequate volume of gas, it is necessary to use a volume-limited ventilator. Consequently, a volume-limited ventilator is more commonly used for continuous mechanical ventilation.

A potential hazard of a volume-limited ventilator is barotrauma. To reduce the risk of pressure-related lung injuries, this type of ventilator is equipped with a pressure-limiting device. The device monitors the airway pressure and vents the system to the atmosphere whenever an established pressure limit is reached. In addition, the device often has an alarm that sounds to alert responsible personnel of the situation. When using a volume-limited ventilator, the monitoring device is ordinarily set to prevent the pressure from exceeding the patient's normal cycling pressure by more than approximately 10 cm H_2O.

During normal breathing, an individual will sigh periodically. The function of the sigh is to prevent the occurrence of microatelectasis. Since a volume ventilator provides a constant tidal volume, this condition can occur unless we are able to provide periodic deep breaths for the patient. The deep breath control or sigh mechanism is usually adjusted to deliver a sigh volume approximately one and one-half times the patient's tidal volume.

It is essential that respiratory care personnel be knowledgeable of the particular ventilator being used. To become familiar with the equipment, the literature provided by the manufacturer should be read and thoroughly understood. In addition, the ventilator should be assembled and attached to a test lung so that various situations, both normal and problem-related, can be simulated. Considerable skill in troubleshooting and correcting problems with ventilator operation should be developed before assuming responsibility for operating the machine for patient care.

Indications and Hazards

A wide variety of physiological and pathological conditions can lead to the need for continuous mechanical ventilation. These conditions include factors that result in mechanical failure of breathing, as well as both primary and secondary disease processes that affect the respiratory system. The presence of these underlying conditions may produce one or more of the following indications for continuous mechanical ventilation.

Indications

The conditions that indicate a need for continuous mechanical ventilation include the following:

1. Apnea, or the complete cessation of breathing, resulting from such conditions as cardiac arrest, drug overdose or pulmonary disorders.

2. Acute respiratory failure as characterized by a pH less than 7.30 and a $PaCO_2$ greater than 60 mmHg, resulting from such conditions as COPD or adult respiratory distress syndrome (ARDS).

3. Inadequate ventilatory reserve as indicated by a tidal volume less than 4 to 5 ml/kg, an FVC less than 10 to 15 ml/kg and an MIP less than -20 cm H_2O, resulting from such conditions as myasthenia gravis or Guillain-Barré syndrome.

4. Severe hypoxemia, characterized by a PaO_2 less than 40 mmHg, resulting from such conditions as pneumonia or noxious gas poisoning.

In summary, the following criteria provide indications for initiating continous mechanical ventilation:

1.   Tidal volume less than 4 to 5 ml/kg

2.   Forced vital capacity less than 10 to 15 ml/kg

3.   MIP less than -20 cm H_2O

4.   pH less than 7.30

5. $PaCO_2$ greater than 60 mmHg

6. PaO_2 less than 40 mmHg

Decisions regarding the initiations of continuous ventilation usually take the overall condition into consideration. This means that each of the previous criteria should be examined and considered collectively when determining the need for ventilatory assistance. Since the patient is subjected to considerable risk during mechanical ventilation, such therapy should only be administered when warranted by the potential benefits. Except in obviously acute situations such as apnea, the potential risks should be thoroughly assessed before initiating continuous mechanical ventilation.

Hazards

There are a number of potential hazards associated with continuous mechanical ventilation. Because this procedure actualy combines several separate procedures or modalities, many of the hazards have been presented in earlier modules. **Table 13-1** on the next page lists the previously described hazards, along with the procedure with which they are associated. Additional hazards associated with continuous mechanical ventilation include:

1.   Inadequate ventilation due to neglecting the responsibility of monitoring blood gas values.

2.   Failure to provide adequate ventilation due to patient disconnect, gross leaks in the system or leakage around the artificial airway cuff.

3.   Equipment failure due to mechanical malfunction of the ventilator, electrical power failure or less-than-adequate supply of source gas.

Table 13-1
Hazards Associated with Component Procedures of Continuous Mechanical Vantilation

Oxygen Delivery	Oxygen-induced hypoventilation Absorption atelectasis Oxygen toxicity
Positive pressure breathing	Hyperventilation Pneumothorax Gastric distention
Medication Delivery	Tachycardia Cardiac arrhythmia Bronchospasm
Artificial airways	Epithelial trauma Tracheal malacia Tracheal stenosis
Tracheal suctioning	Mucosal damage Cardiac arrhythmia Bradycardia Hypotension Infection Atelectasis

4. Infection due to immunosuppression and failure of personnel to maintain asepsis while handling equipment and performing routine ventilator maintenance and patient care procedures.

5. Decreased venous return and cardiac output due to increased intrathoracic pressure exerted by the gas delivered under positive pressure.

6. Gastrointestinal bleeding and ulcers created by the stress associated with the extended use of continuous mechanical ventilation.

Table 13-1.
Hazards associated
with component
procedures of
continuous mechani-
cal ventilation.

Patient Monitoring

Patients receiving continuous mechanical ventilation in the intensive care unit must be closely monitored. This monitoring should include a complete ventilator check at least every two hours and at least daily assessment of the adequacy of ventilation and ventilatory reserve. Changes in the patient's condition may indicate a need for more frequent assessment of ventilatory status.

The most accurate method of assessing the adequacy of ventilation is to perform a blood gas analysis. If the blood gas values deviate from the normal range for the patient, thus indicating inadequacy of ventilation, the physician should be contacted immediately. The ventilatory reserve is monitored routinely to detect changes in the degree of ventilatory assistance needed by the patient. The purpose and procedure for performing the periodic ventilator checks are discussed in a subsequent section of this module.

Respiratory care personnel should be mindful of the fact that the patient has many needs other than adequacy of ventilation. Because of the emotional trauma associated with continuous ventilation, it is important to provide comfort and assurance to the patient. This includes carefully explaining procedures to be performed and attempting to maintain two-way communication, as well as offering words of encouragement and reassurance. It is equally important to avoid insensitive comments and conversation in the presence of the patient, even one who is comatose. Always remember that the patient is more than just another ventilator attachment.

Clinical Procedure 13.1
Ventilator Set Up

Patients are usually placed on a ventilator in emergency situations. Since it is nearly impossible to predict in advance when a ventilator will be needed, it is advisable to have at least one standby ventilator ready for use at all times. The standby ventilator should be completely assembled, except for placing water in the humidifier, and tested to ensure that it functions properly. The standby ventilator should be covered and stored in a convenient location close to the patient care area. If the ventilator is not used within three days, the equipment should be changed and the testing process repeated.

A ventilator set up must be checked for proper function, for leaks in the circuit, and for accurate control of oxygen delivery according to specific guidelines developed by the manufacturer. When searching for leaks in a ventilator circuit, it is recommended that a systematic procedure be followed. Starting at the ventilator outlet, each connection in the path of the gas flow is checked in turn. If no leaks have been found by the time the spirometer is reached, the problem may be with the spirometer itself.

Testing for the accurate control of oxygen delivery can be done by placing a calibrated oxygen analyzer in the circuit to measure the actual concentration of the oxygen delivered during operation. With the oxygen control set at 40% and the ventilator operating at a rate above 10 breaths per minute, the analyzer should register $40 \pm 3\%$ within two minutes. While waiting for the oxygen to achieve a consistent reading, all lights and alarms should be checked to assure proper working order. Any ventilator malfunction that cannot be readily corrected by minor adjustments or replacement of parts will necessitate obtaining and assembling another machine.

Procedure for Performing a Ventilator Set Up

The following procedure is recommended for setting up a standby ventilator:

A. *Maintain Asepsis.* While performing the remainder of this procedure, you are expected to maintain aseptic conditions according to the procedures described in **SSE 1.2**. This includes washing your hands:

   • Before obtaining equipment
   • Following performance of **D. Test Equipment**
   • Anytime during the procedure that contamination is suspected

B. *Obtain Equipment.* Collect the following equipment and supplies:

- Volume ventilator
- Ventilator circuit
- Spirometer (as applicable)
- Humidifier
- Flex tube
- Oxygen analyzer
- Test lung
- Temperature probe
- Patient attachment
- Resuscitation bag and mask
- Filters
- Condensor vial (if applicable)
- High-pressure hose(s) and gas-source connector(s)
- Water traps

C. *Assemble Equipment.* Prepare the equipment for use as follows:

1. Insert the filters. (Type and positioning of filters varies with ventilator brands).

2. Connect the humidifier to the ventilator. (Since this is a standby ventilator, do not fill the humidifier with water.)

3. Connect the flex tube or humidifier adaptor between the humidifier inlet and the ventilator outlet.

4. Attach the inspiratory tubing of the ventilator tubing circuit to the humidifier outlet.

5. Attach the expiratory tubing of the ventilator circuit to the ventilator or the spirometer (whichever is applicable).

6. Connect the exhalation valve tubing. (as applicable)

7. If applicable, connect the spirometer tubing to the spirometer outlet.

8. If applicable, connect the proximal airway pressure line.

9. Insert the temperature probe into the inspiratory tubing of the ventilator circuit.

10. Connect the test lung to the patient attachment.

11. Connect the high-pressure hose(s) to the gas inlet(s) on the ventilator.

12. If applicable, connect auxiliary alarms to the inspiratory tubing of the ventilator circuit.

D. ***Test Equipment.*** Test the ventilator equipment as follows:

1. Connect the ventilator to the electrical and gas outlets.

2. Turn all controls off.

3. Set the volume control at 500 ml.

4. Set the pressure limit control above 20 cm H_2O.

5. To test for leaks, manually cycle the ventilator.

6. If the spirometer or exhaled gas monitor does not register 500 ml ($\pm$10) after five cycles, tighten all connections and repeat.

7. If the spirometer still does not register 500 ml, check for leaks by inserting a portable spirometer in each connection of the gas flow pathway.

8. If no leak is found, replace the spirometer.

9. If the spirometer still does not register 500 ml:

    a. Lable the ventilator as "defective" and replace it.

    b. Reassemble and retest the new equipment.

10. Set the oxygen control at 40% and the respiratory rate above 10 breaths per minute.

11. Place a calibrated oxygen analyzer to assure proper working order. Make minor adjustments as necessary.

12. Test all lights and alarms to assure proper working order. Make minor adjustments as necessary.

13. If, within two minutes, the analyzer does not register 40 $\pm$ 3%:

    a. Lable the ventilator as "defective" and replace it.

    b. Reassemble and retest the new equipment.

14. Cover the ventilator and store it in a convenient location.

Clinical Procedure 13.2
Ventilator Check

During operation, a mechanical ventilator should be checked at least every one to two hours to ensure proper functioning. This check includes repeating test procedures similar to those performed at the time the ventilator was set up. In addition, it is necessary to check and make appropriate adjustments to ensure that the ventilator control parameters match the physician's order, that the gas temperature is at or near body temperature and that the humidifier contains sufficient water. It is also necessary to drain the accumulated condensate from the ventilator circuit and water traps without allowing it to return to the humidifier.

In conjunction with the ventilator check, the patient's status must also be assessed. This includes evaluating the patient's appearance, auscultating the chest, checking vital signs, suctioning the airway as necessary and measuring pulmonary compliance. Any changes in the patient's status should be noted and the physician notified if the patient's condition appears unstable.

Procedure for Performing a Ventilator Check

It is recommended that a ventilator check be performed according to the following procedure:

A. *Maintain Asepsis.* While performing the remainder of this procedure, you are expected to maintain aseptic conditions and follow universal precautions according to the procedures described in **SSE 1.2**. This includes washing your hands:

    • Before obtaining equipment
    • Following performance of *G. Test Equipment*
    • Anytime during the procedure that contamination is suspected

B. *Obtain Equipment.* Collect the following equipment and supplies:

    • Stethoscope
    • Portable spirometer with patient attachment
    • Oxygen analyzer
    • Suction equipment

C. *Confirm Patient.* Ensure that the procedure is performed with the correct patient as follows:

1. Match the information on the order with the following:

   • Room number
   • Name on the door or bed
   • Name on the wristband

2. Greet the patient by name (in a questioning manner if unknown).

3. Resolve any discrepancies in the patient identification information by conferring with the nursing staff.

D. *Inform Patient.* Interact with the patient as follows:

1. Introduce yourself by name and department (if not already acquainted).

2. Tell the patient what procedure is to be performed.

3. Explain the procedure by describing:

   • Why it is to be performed
   • How it will be performed
   • What the patient is expected to do
   • What you will be doing
   • How frequently it will be performed

E. *Implement Procedure.* Perform the following tasks:

1. Assess the patient's appearance regarding color, state of consciousness and comfort. Record the results.

2. *Empty Condensate.* Empty any condensate present from the ventilator tubing, moving water away from the patient and into the appropriate reservoir (i.e., wastebasket, water traps, etc.; *not* the humidifier).

3. *Wash hands.* Wash your hands according to the procedure described in **SSE 1.1**.

4. *Auscultate Chest.* Auscultate the patient's chest according to the procedure described in **SSE 2.2**. If adventitious sounds are audible, suction the patient according to the procedure described in **CPE 12.1**.

5. *Check Pulse.* Count the heart rate for at least one minute. Record results.

6. *Check Respiratory Rate.* Compare the respiratory rate ordered by the physician with the patient's actual respiratory rate. Record the results.

7. *Check Tidal Volume.* Compare the tidal volume ordered by the physician with the tidal volume exhaled. If necessary, adjust the volume in order to maintain the tidal volume ordered by the physician. Record the results.

8. *Check Sigh Volume.* Manually sigh the patient to compare the sigh volume ordered by the physician with the sigh volume exhaled. Record the results.

9. *Analyze FIO_2.* If necessary, adjust the inspired oxygen concentration in order to maintain the FIO_2 ordered by the physician. Record the results.

10. *Check Flow Rate.* If necessary, adjust the flow rate to maintain an I:E ratio of at least 1:1½ or the ratio ordered by the physician. Record the results.

11. *Check Pressure Limit.* Compare the system pressure limit with the patient's airway pressure. Adjust as necessary to maintain a system pressure limit of 10 cm H_2O above the airway pressure.

12. *Check Static Compliance.* Subtract the PEEP pressure from the plateau pressure and divide the tidal volume received by the difference. Record the results.

13. *Check Temperature.* Check the temperature of the inspired gas and, if necessary, adjust the heater in order to obtain a temperature of $98 \pm 2°F$. Record the results.

14. *Check Alarms.* Check the operation of all alarms to assure that all lights, fuses and/or batteries are functioning properly.

15. *Check Other Parameters.* Check any applicable parameters (i.e., PEEP, IMV, sensitivity, etc.). Record the results.

16. *Check Humidifier.* Check the water level of the humidifier and add sterile water if needed.

17. *Auscultate Chest.* Auscultate the patient's chest according to the procedure described in **SSE 2.2.** If adventitious sounds are

audible, suction the patient according to the procedure described in **CPE 12.1**.

F. *Record Information.* Document the ventilator check as follows:

1. Record the following:

   • Breath sounds
   • Sputum volume, color, and consistency
   • Other pertinent information

2. Make certain that all of the following results obtained in Steps 1 through 15 were recorded clearly:

   • Pulse rate
   • Respiratory rate(s)
   • Tidal volume
   • Sigh volume
   • FIO_2
   • Flow rate
   • System pressure
   • Static compliance
   • Temperature
   • Other applicable parameters

G. *Conclude Procedure.* Complete the following tasks:

1. Place the patient in a comfortable position.

2. Assure that the call bell and bedside table are within the patient's reach.

3. Ask if the patient has any needs. (Many patients on ventilators can effectively communicate by writing or pointing to pictures.)

4. Answer any questions as effectively as possible.

H. *Report Observations.* Report the following information:

1. Reportany significant adverse changes in the patient's condition to the nurse or physician whenever observed.

2. Following the procedure, inform the appropriate personnel of:

   • Patient requests
   • Patient complaints
   • Unexpressed patient needs

3. Following the procedure, report to the nurse or physician:

    • Any non-critical adverse reactions to the therapy
    • Other pertinent observations of the patient's condition

Clinical Procedure 13.3
Ventilator Change-Out

Infection poses a serious risk for patients receiving mechanical ventilation. In order to reduce contamination and minimize the risk of infection, the ventilator circuit should be changed at least every 24 to 48 hours. This procedure involves replacement of all removal parts of the ventilator circuit which come in contact with the patient's inhaled or exhaled air. Since the patient is dependent upon the ventilator for breathing assistance, it is important that this procedure be performed quickly and efficiently. This can best be accomplished by assembling and changing-out entire sections of the circuitry at a time. Once the ventilator change-out is complete, a ventilator check should be performed to ensure that the ventilator is still functioning properly.

Procedure for Performing a Ventilator Change-Out

A. *Maintain Asepsis.* While performing the remainder of this procedure, you are expected to maintain aseptic conditions and follow universal precautions according to the procedures described in **SSE 1.2**. This includes washing your hands:

- Before obtaining equipment
- Following performance of *F. Conclude Procedure*
- Anytime during the procedure that contamination is suspected

B. *Obtain Equipment.* Collect the following equipment and supplies:

- Ventilator circuit and manifold
- Spirometer
- Humidifier
- Sterile water
- Flex tube
- Temperature probe
- Patient attachment
- Water traps
- Filters
- Oxygen analyzer
- Stethoscope

C. *Confirm Patient.* Ensure that the procedure is performed with the correct patient as follows:

1. Match the information on the order with the following:

   - Room number
   - Name on the door or bed
   - Name on the wristband

2. Greet the patient by name (in a questioning manner if unknown).

3. Resolve any discrepancies in the patient identification information by conferring with the nursing staff.

D. ***Inform Patient.*** Interact with the patient as follows:

1. Introduce yourself by name and department (if not already acquainted).

2. Tell the patient what procedure is to be performed.

3. Explain the procedure by describing:

   - Why it is to be performed
   - How it will be performed
   - What the patient is expected to do
   - What you will be doing
   - How frequently it will be performed

E. ***Implement Procedure.*** Perform the following tasks:

1. *Remove Humidifier.* Bypass the humidifier by connecting the inlet tubing of the ventilator circuit directly to the ventilator outlet.

2. *Replace Humidifier.* Attach the clean humidifier (filled with sterile water) to the heating element.

3. *Disconnect Used Outlet Tubing.* Remove the used outlet tubing of the ventilator circuit from either the condensor vial or the spirometer (whichever is applicable).

4. *Connect Ventilator Circuit.* Attach the inlet tubing of the ventilator circuit to either the clean condensor vial or the clean spirometer (whichever is applicable).

5. *Sigh Patient.* In preparation for disconnection from the ventilator, give the patient several deep breaths by either pressing the manual sigh button or by temporarily increasing the tidal volume and pressing the manual breath button.

6. *Change Circuits*. Connect the patient to the clean circuitry as follows:

   a. Disconnect the used ventilator circuit from the ventilator outlet and replace it with the flex tube attached to the clean humidifier.

   b. Disconnect the used exhalation valve tubing and replace it with the clean exhalation valve tubing.

   c. Disconnect the used ventilator circuit from the patient and replace it with the clean ventilator circuit.

   (**Note:** These steps should take no longer than 15 seconds.)

7. *Sigh Patient*. Repeat the sigh maneuver.

8. *Perform Ventilator Check*. Perform a ventilator check according to the procedure described in **CPE 13.2**.

9. *Change Filters*. Change the filters according to the manufacturer's specifications.

F.   ***Conclude Procedure***. Complete the following tasks:

1. Place the patient in a comfortable position.

2. Assure that the call bell and bedside table are within the patient's reach.

3. Ask if the patient has any needs. (Many patients on ventilators can effectively communicate by writing or pointing to pictures.)

4. Answer any questions as effectively as possible.

G.   ***Report Observations***. Report the following information:

1. Report any significant adverse changes in the patient's condition to the nurse or physician whenever observed.

2. Following the procedure, inform the appropriate personnel of:

   • Patient requests
   • Patient complaints
   • Unexpressed patient needs

3. Following the procedure, report to the nurse or physician:

   • Any non-critical adverse reactions to the therapy
   • Other pertinent observations of the patient's condition

Clinical Procedure 13.4
Positive End-Expiratory Pressure

Normal alveoli remain slightly expanded at the end of expiration which means that a small volume of gas always remains. If the volume of retained gas drops below a critical minimum level, elastic forces will cause the alveoli to collapse, thus reducing the residual volume and therefore the functional residual capacity (FRC). This collapse of alveoli results in the occurrence of shunting and subsequent hypoxemia. In addition, pulmonary compliance is decreased because alveolar collapse requires increased pressure to inflate the lungs. This condition greatly increases the work of breathing necessary for a patient to maintain alveolar ventilation.

It is possible to maintain sufficient pressure within the system during continuous mechanical ventilation to prevent the patient's FRC from dropping below the critical volume. The procedure in which the intrathoracic pressure is not allowed to return to atmospheric pressure during expiration is known as positive end-expiratory pressure (PEEP). In addition to increasing the FRC, PEEP reduces the risk of oxygen toxicity because adequate arterial oxygenation can be maintained at a lower FIO_2. Because PEEP increases intrathoracic pressure, however, it has the potential of causing hypotension, decreased cardiac output and pneumothorax.

Procedure for Providing PEEP

Whenever ordered during continuous mechanical ventilation, PEEP should be provided according to the following procedure:

A. *Check Order.* Verify the physician's order as follows:

   1. Compare the requisition with the physician's order to ensure that no discrepancies exist.

   2. Review the order to ensure that the following are prescribed:

      • Level of PEEP
      • Patient's ventilator control mode (assist, assist-control or control)

   3. If any part of the order is unfamiliar, question its accuracy.

B. *Review Chart.* Use the following procedure to review the patient's chart:

1. On the patient's chart, identify all pertinent data in the following areas.

   - History and physical
   - Admitting diagnosis
   - Progress notes
   - Blood gas analysis
   - Chest x-ray

2. Based on the patient data, identify the following:

C. *Maintain Asepsis.* While performing the remainder of this procedure, you are expected to maintain aseptic conditions and follow universal precautions according to the procedure described in **SSE 1.2**. This includes washing your hands:

- Before obtaining equipment
- Following performance of **H. Conclude Procedure**
- Anytime during the procedure that contamination is suspected

D. *Obtain Equipment.* Collect the following equipment and supplies:

- PEEP attachment (if not already connected)
- Stethoscope
- Sphygmomanometer

E. *Confirm Patient.* Ensure that the procedure is performed with the correct patient as follows:

1. Match the information on the order with the following:

   - Room number
   - Name on the door or bed
   - Name on the wristband

2. Greet the patient by name (in a questioning manner if unknown).

3. Resolve any discrepancies in the patient identification information by conferring with the nursing staff.

F. *Inform Patient.* Interact with the patient as follows:

1. Introduce yourself by name and department (if not already acquainted).

2. Tell the patient what procedure is to be performed.

3. Explain the procedure by describing:

   - Why it is to be performed
   - How it will be performed
   - What the patient is expected to do
   - What you will be doing
   - How frequently it will be performed

G. **Implement Procedure.** Perform the following tasks:

   1. *Perform Ventilator Check.* Perform a ventilator check according to the procedure described in **CPE 13.2.**

   2. *Monitor Blood Pressure.* Measure and record the patient's blood pressure.

   3. *Adjust Controls.* Adjust the following controls as needed:

      - PEEP valve (to desired PEEP level)
      - System pressure limit (10 cm H_2O above the patient's air way pressure)
      - Sensitivity control (if assisting respirations)

   4. *Perform Ventilator Check.* Perform ventilator check according to the procedure described in **CPE 13.2.**

   5. *Monitor Blood Pressure.* Measure and record the patient's blood pressure. Notify the appropriate personnel if the patient's blood pressure falls more than 10%.

H. **Conclude Procedure.** Complete the following tasks:

   1. Place the patient in a comfortable position.

   2. Assure that the call bell and bedside table are within the patient's reach.

   3. Ask if the patient has any needs.

   4. Answer any questions as effectively as possible.

I. **Report Observations.** Report the following information:

   1. Report any significant adverse changes in the patient's condition to the nurse or physician whenever observed.

2. Following the procedure, inform the appropriate personnel of

   - Patient requests
   - Patient complaints
   - Unexpressed patient needs

3. Following the procedure, report to the nurse or physician:

   - Any non-critical adverse reactions to the therapy
   - Other pertinent observations of the patient's condition

Clinical Procedure 13.5
Intermittent Mandatory Ventilation

Intermittent mandatory ventilation (IMV) is a procedure that combines positive pressure breathing with spontaneous unassisted breathing. With this procedure, a mechanical ventilator continues to provide mandatory breaths at regular predetermined intervals. When the patient attempts to breathe spontaneously, however, instead of cycling the ventilator, an adjunct circuit provides gas at atmospheric pressure for spontaneous ventilation. By gradually reducing the frequency of the mandatory breaths, the patient is encouraged to take more spontaneous breaths. Therefore, IMV is especially suitable for weaning the patient from a ventilator.

The administration of IMV tends to minimize patient dependence on a mechanical ventilator. It also tends to reduce any anxiety associated with abrupt discontinuance of mechanical ventilation. In addition, IMV enables the patient to improve muscular strength in order to regain control of respiration and regulation of blood gases. For these reasons, it is recommended that IMV be admininstered to all patients who are capable of occasional unassisted breathing, particularly during the period of ventilator discontinuance.

There are several ways of providing intermittent mandatory ventilation for a ventilator patient. Most ventilators is use today are equipped with IMV capability. Earlier models require the use of ancillary equipment. The procedures used to administer IMV are usually determined by the type of equipment available in the hospital. No matter how the procedure is performed, an adequate flow rate and relative humidity must be provided at the same FIO_2 as delivered by the ventilator. If it is necessary to deliver IMV by means of ancillary equipment, the following procedure is recommended.

Procedure for Providing IMV

Whenever ordered as an ancillary procedure during continuous mechanical ventilation, IMV should be provided in the following manner:

A.   *Check Order.* Verify the physician's order as follows:

1.   Compare the requisition with the physician's order to ensure that no discrepancies exist.

2.   Review the order to ascertain the IMV rate.

3. If any part of the order is unfamiliar, question its accuracy.

B. ***Review Chart.*** Use the following procedure to review the patient's chart:

1. On the patient's chart, identify all pertinent data in the following areas:

   • History and physical
   • Admitting diagnosis
   • Progress notes
   • Blood gas analysis
   • Chest x-ray

2. Based on the patient data, identify the benefits of IMV.

C. ***Maintain Asepsis.*** While performing the remainder of this procedure, you are expected to maintain aseptic conditions and observe universal precautions according to the procedure described in **SSE 1.2**. This includes washing your hands:

• Before obtaining equipment
• Following performance of ***J. Conclude Procedure***
• Anytime during the procedure that contamination is suspected

D. ***Obtain Equipment.*** Collect the following equipment and supplies:

• IMV "H" valve
• Aerosol nebulizer with heater
• Sterile water or normal saline
• Three mainstream hoses
• Low-flow oxygen blender
• Oxygen analyzer

E. ***Assemble Equipment.*** Prepare the equipment for use as follows:

1. Fill the nebulizer to the fill line with sterile water or normal saline.

2. Connect one mainstream hose between the aerosol outlet and the "H" valve (Port 1).

3. Attach another mainstream hose to the "H" valve (Port 2).

4. Attach the third mainstream hose to the "H" valve (Port 3).

5. Connect the oxygen blender to the aerosol nebulizer (See **Figure 13.1**.)

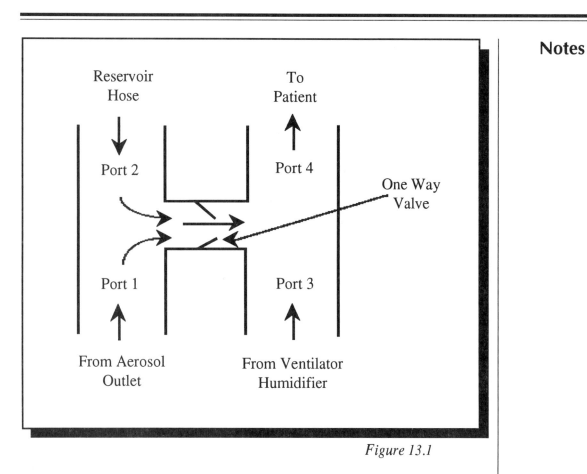

Figure 13.1

F. ***Test Equipment.*** Test the equipment as follows:

1. Test the aerosol equipment according to the procedure described in **CPE 10.1**.

2. Ensure that the one-way valve in the "H" valve moves freely.

3. Adjust the oxygen concentration to match the value appearing on the order.

G. ***Confirm Patient.*** Ensure that the procedure is performed with the correct patient as follows:

1. Match the information on the order with the following:

   • Room number
   • Name on the door or bed
   • Name on the wristband

2. Greet the patient by name (in a questioning manner if unknown).

3. Resolve any discrepancies in the patient identification information by conferring with the nursing staff.

H. *Inform Patient.* Interact with the patient as follows:

1. Introduce yourself by name and department (if not already acquainted).

2. Tell the patient what procedure is to be performed.

3. Explain the procedure by describing:

   • Why it is to be performed
   • How it will be performed
   • What the patient is expected to do
   • What you will be doing
   • How frequently it will be performed

I. *Implement Procedure.* Perform the following tasks:

1. *Perform Ventilator Check.* Perform a ventilator check according to the procedure described in **CPE 13.2**.

2. *Attach IMV Set Up.* Perform the following steps:

   a. Connect the oxygen blender to the gas outlet.

   b. Disconnect the inlet tubing of the ventilator circuit from the humidifier outlet.

   c. Attach the mainstream tubing connected to Port 3 of the "H" valve to the humidifier outlet.

   d. Connect the inlet tubing to the "H" valve (Port 4).

   e. Set the oxygen blender flow rate above 10 liters per minute.

3. *Adjust Controls.* Adjust the following controls as necessary:

   • Adjust the mandatory rate to match the physician's order
   • Turn off the sensitivity control

4. *Analyze FIO_2.* Analyze the FIO_2 and adjust, as necessary, to ensure that the FIO_2 matches the value appearing on the order.

5. *Perform Ventilator Check.* Perform ventilator check according to the procedure described in **CPE 13.2**.

J. *Conclude Procedure.* Complete the following tasks:

1. Place the patient in a comfortable position.

2. Assure that the call bell and bedside table are within the patient's reach.

3. Ask if the patient has any needs.

4. Answer any questions as effectively as possible.

K. *Report Observations.* Report the following information:

1. Report any significant adverse changes in the patient's condition to the nurse or physician whenever observed.

2. Following the procedure, inform the appropriate personnel of

   • Patient requests
   • Patient complaints
   • Unexpressed patient needs

3. Following the procedure, report to the nurse or physician:

   • Any non-critical adverse reactions to the therapy
   • Other pertinent observations of the patient's condition

Evaluation of Ventilator Management Procedures

The following definitions are provided for use whenever the respective Ventilator Management Procedures are evaluated. In order for performance of the procedures to be considered acceptable, all Essential Tasks must be performed according to the accompanying Evaluation Criteria. Any deviation from the following task sequence or criteria must be approved by the evaluator.

CPE 13.1 Ventilator Set Up		
Performance	**Essential Tasks**	**Evaluation Criteria**
A. Maintain Asepsis	See SSE 1.2	See SSE 1.2
B. Obtain Equipment	1. Obtains the following equipment and supplies: • Volume ventilator • Ventilator circuit and manifold • Spirometer • Humidifier • Flex tube • Oxygen analyzer • Test lung • Temperature probe • Patient attachment • Condensor vial (if applicable) • Filters • Resuscitation bag and mask • High pressure hose(s) and gas source connectors	a. Correct equipment obtained
C. Assemble Equipment	1. Prepares equipment as follows: • Filters inserted • Humidifier connected • Circuit connected to ventilator • Spirometer connected • Temperature probe inserted • Test lung attached • Auxilliary alarms connected (if applicable)	a. Assembled according to **SOP**

CPE 13.1		
Ventilator Set Up (continued)		
Performance	**Essential Tasks**	**Evaluation Criteria**
D. Test Equipment	1. Tests for: • Functioning of spirometer • Functioning of oxygen blender • Functioning of alarms • Leaks in System	a. Tested according to **SOP** b. Leaks remedied c. Defective equipment replaced

CPE 13.2 Ventilator Check		
Performance	**Essential Tasks**	**Evaluation Criteria**
A. Maintain Asepsis	See **SSE 1.2**	See **SSE 1.2**
B. Obtain Equipment	1. Obtains the following equipment and supplies: • Stethoscope • Portable spirometer • Oxygen analyzer • Suction equipment	a. Correct equipment obtained
C. Confirm Patient	See **SSE 3.3**	See **SSE 1.2**
D. Inform Patient	See **SSE 4.1**	See **SSE 4.1**
E. Implement Procedure	1. Determines the following patient characteristics: • Color • State of consciousness • Agitation	a. Assessed correctly
	2. Empties condensate	a. Emptied away from patient b. Emptied into appropriate reservoir (not humidifier)
	3. Washes hands	a. Performed according to **SSE 1.1**
	4. Auscultates chest	a. Performed according to **SSE 2.2**
	5. Checks pulse	a. Counted for at least one (1) minute b. Results recorded
	6. Checks respiratory rate	a. Counted for at least one (1) minute b. Actual value compared with ordered value c. Results recorded

CPE 13.2
Ventilator Check (continued)

Performance	Essential Tasks	Evaluation Criteria
E. Implement Procedure (continued)	7. Checks tidal volume	a. Exhaled tidal volume compared with order b. Tidal volume adjusted when necessary c. Results recorded
	8. Checks sigh volume	a. Exhaled sigh volume compared with order b. Sigh volume adjusted when necessary c. Results recorded
	9. Analyzes FIO_2	a. FIO_2 being administeredcompared with order b. FIO_2 adjusted when necessary to match order c. Results recorded
	10. Checks flow rate	a. I:E ratio compared with order. b. I:E ratio adjusted when necessary to maintain 1:1 $^1/_2$, or as ordered c. Results recorded
	11. Checks system pressure limit	a. System pressure compared with patient's airway pressure b. System pressure adjusted to 10 cm H_2O (or less) above airway pressure
	12. Checks static compliance	a. PEEP subtracted from plateau pressure b. Tidal volume divided by difference c. Results recorded
	13. Checks temperature	a. Inspired gas temperature measured. b. Heater adusted to maintain temperature of $98 \pm 2°$ (if necessary)
	14. Checks alarms	a. Functioning of lights assured b. Functioning of fuses and/or batteries assured
	15. Checks other parameters: • PEEP • IMV • Sensitivity	a. Parameters adjusted as necessary b. Results recorded

CPE 13.2
Ventilator Check (continued)

Performance	Essential Tasks	Evaluation Criteria
E. Implement Procedure (continued)	16. Checks humidifier	a. Water level checked b. Sterile water added if necessary
	17. Auscultates chest	a. Performed according to SSE 2.2 b. Patient suctioned if adventitious sounds are audible
F. Record Information	1. Records the following patient data: • Breath sounds • Sputum volume • Sputum consistency • Sputum color • Other pertinent information.	a. Only factual information recorded b. No important details omitted c. No irrelevant data recorded d. All information accurate e. All errors properly corrected
	2. Assures that the following results are recorded: • Pulse rate • Respiratory rate(s) • Tidal volume • Sigh volume • FIO$_2$ • Flow rate • System pressure • Static compliance • Temperature • Other applicable parameters.	a. Only factual information recorded b. No important details omitted c. No irrelevant data recorded d. All information accurate e. All errors properly corrected
G. Conclude Procedure	1. Replaces call bell and bedside table	a. Placed within patient's reach
	2. Tends to patient needs	a. Comfortable position assured b. Patient asked regarding other needs c. Patient questions answered effectively
H. Report Observations	See SSE 4.3	See SSE 4.3

CPE 13.3 Ventilator Change-Out		
Performance	**Essential Tasks**	**Evaluation Criteria**
A. Maintain Asepsis	See **SSE 1.2**	See **SSE 1.2**
B. Obtain Equipment	1. Obtains the following equipment and supplies: • Ventilator circuit and manifold. • Spirometer • Humidifier • Sterile water • Flex tube • Temperature probe • Patient attachment • Condensor vial (if applicable) • Filters • Oxygen analyzer • Stethoscope	a. Correct equipment obtained
C. Confirm Patient	See **SSE 3.3**	See **SSE 1.2**
D. Inform Patient	See **SSE 4.1**	See **SSE 4.1**
E. Implement Procedure	1. Performs ventilator check	a. Performed according to **CPE 13.2**
	2. Removes humidifier	a. Humidifier bypassed
	3. Replaces humidifier	a. Clean humidifier attached to heating element b. Sterile water added
	4. Disconnects used outlet tubing	a. Tubing removed
	5. Connects ventilator circuit.	a. Inlet tubing connected to humidifier b. Outlet tubing connected to either spirometer or condensor vial (whichever is applicable)
	6. Sighs patient	a. Manual deep breaths provided

	CPE 13.3 Ventilator Change-Out (continued)	
Performance	**Essential Tasks**	**Evaluation Criteria**
E. Implement Procedure (continued)	7. Changes circuit	a. Clean humidifier placed in line b. Exhalation valve tubing replaced c. Patient connected to clean ventilator circuit
	8. Sighs patient	a. Manual deep breaths provided
	9. Performs ventilator check	a. Performed according to **CPE 13.2**
	10. Changes filters	a. Changed according to manufacturer's specifications
F. Conclude Procedure	1. Replaces call bell and bedside table	a. Placed within patient's reach
	2. Tends to patient needs	a. Comfortable position assured b. Patient asked regarding other needs c. Patient questions answered effectively
G. Report Observations	See **SSE 4.3**	See **SSE 4.3**

CPE 13.4
Positive End-Expiratory Pressure

Performance	Essential Tasks	Evaluation Criteria
A. Check Order	See SSE 3.1	See SSE 3.1
B. Review Chart	See SSE 3.2	See SSE 3.2
C. Maintain Asepsis	See SSE 1.2	See SSE 1.2
D. Obtain Equipment	1. Obtains the following equipment and supplies: • PEEP attachment (if not already attached) • Stethoscope • Sphygmomanometer	a. Correct equipment obtained
E. Confirm Patient	See SSE 3.3	See SSE 3.3
F. Inform Patient	See SSE 4.1	See SSE 4.1
G. Implement Procedure	1. Performs ventilator check	a. Performed according to CPE 13.2
	2. Monitors blood pressure	a. Procedure performed correctly
	3. Adjusts controls	a. PEEP adjusted to desired level b. System pressure limit set at 10 cm H_2O above airway pressure c. Sensitivity adjusted (if assisting)
	4. Performs ventilator check	a. Performed according to CPE 13.2
	5. Monitors blood pressure	a. Procedure performed correctly b. Personnel notified if blood pressure fell more than 10% c. Results recorded

CPE 13.4 Positive End-Expiratory Pressure (continued)		
Performance	**Essential Tasks**	**Evaluation Criteria**
H. Conclude Procedure	1. Replaces call bell and bedside table	a. Placed within patient's reach
	2. Tends to patient needs	a. Comfortable position assured b. Patient asked regarding other needs c. Patient questions answered effectively
I. Report Observations	See **SSE 4.3**	See **SSE 4.3**

	CPE 13.5	
	Intermittent Mandatory Ventilation	
Performance	**Essential Tasks**	**Evaluation Criteria**
A. Check Order	See **SSE 3.1**	See **SSE 3.1**
B. Review Chart	See **SSE 3.2**	See **SSE 3.2**
C. Maintain Asepsis	See **SSE 1.2**	See **SSE 1.2**
D. Obtain Equipment	1. Obtains the following equipment and supplies: • IMV "H" valve • Aerosol nebulizer with heater • Sterile water or normal saline • 3 mainstream hoses • Low flow oxygen blender • Oxygen analyzer.	a. Correct equipment obtained (if not part of the ventilator)
E. Assemble	1. Prepares equipment as follows: • Fills nebulizer • Connects "H" valves • Connects blender	a. Nebulizer filled with sterile water or saline b. Assembled according to **SOP**
F. Test Equipment	1. Tests for: • Functioning of aerosol • Oxygen concentration	a. Tested according to **SOP** b. Leaks remedied c. Defective equipment replaced
G. Confirm Patient	See **SSE 3.3**	See **SSE 3.3**
H. Inform Patient	See **SSE 4.1**	See **SSE 4.1**
I. Implement Procedure	1. Performs ventilator check 2. Attaches IMV set up	a. Performed according to **CPE 13.2** a. Blender connected to gas outlet b. Ventilator circuit inlet tubing connected to the open port on "H" valve

CPE 13.5
Intermittent Mandatory Ventilation (continued)

Performance	Essential Tasks	Evaluation Criteria
I. Implement Procedure (continued)		c. "H" valve connected to humidifier d. Blender flow rate set above 10 lpm
	3. Adjusts controls	a. Correct IMV rate established. b. Sensitivity turned off
	4. Analyzes FIO_2	a. FIO_2 adjusted to match order
	5. Performs ventilator check	a. Performed according to **CPE 13.2**
J. Conclude Procedure	1. Replaces call bell and bedside table	a. Placed within patient's reach
	2. Tends to patient needs	a. Comfortable position assured b. Patient asked regarding other needs c. Patient questions answered effectively
K. Report Observations	See **SSE 4.3**	See **SSE 4.3**

Module 14.0

Oxygen Therapy for Infants

Respiratory care of the neonate ranges from the administration of oxygen at ambient pressures to continuous mechanical ventilation. The mode of therapy prescribed depends upon the severity of the infant's respiratory distress. This module presents the administration of oxygen therapy to neonates using either the infant hood or the infant halo as the delivery device.

Objectives

Upon completion of this module, you will be able to:

1. List and explain the conditions that indicate the use of oxygen therapy for an infant.

2. List and describe the potential hazards associated with oxygen therapy.

3. Administer oxygen to an infant by means of an infant hood and halo.

The most common devices for administering oxygen to an infant are the hood, halo, and incubator. The hood and halo have become the preferred devices because they are the simplest methods of delivering a constant FIO_2. In comparison to the incubator, they are much less cumbersome and they allow greater access to the patient. When administering routine nursing care, wide variations in FIO_2 are less likely because the oxygen environment can remain uninterrupted as long as the delivery device is not disturbed.

Clinical Procedure 14.1
Infant Hood or Halo

The oxygen hood is a small plastic covering that fits over the infant's head. A large horseshoe opening at one end fits around the neck and a smaller opening at the other end allows for humidified or aerosolized oxygen to enter via large-bore tubing. Some hoods employ a removable lid or cover to allow easy access to the infant's head, while others are made of a single "bubble" of clear plastic. A halo is essentially an infant hood without the lid. Infant hoods and halos usually employ a heated humdifier or low output nebulizer to avoid cooling of the infant, thereby minimizing oxygen consumption and preventing water loss and secretion dehydration.

Indications

Oxygen therapy is administered to infants and neonates for the treatment of hypoxemia. The most common causes of this condition are atelectasis, pneumonia, and cardiac abnormalities. Whenever the desired effects can be obtained, the preferred method of treating hypoxemia in the infant is by the administration of oxygen at ambient pressure.

Hazards and Precautions

The hazards associated with oxygen therapy for an infant are essentially the same as for adults. An additional concern is the possibility of retinopathy of prematurity caused by *high partial pressures of oxygen in arterial blood*. Frequent monitoring of blood gases and continuous transcutaneous PO_2 or pulse oximetry, is necessary to ensure an adequate supply of oxygen at the lowest possible FIO_2.

The oxygen hood and halo should be closely monitored to make certain that there is not too much condensation within the hood or in the large-bore tubing. There is always the danger of overhydrating the infant when using high humidity or aerosol. In addition, a thermometer should be placed in the hood to aid in the detection of temperature increases which may have an adverse effect on the infant.

Procedure for Administering Oxygen Therapy to Infants

A. *Check Order.* Verify the physician's order as follows:

1. Compare the requisition with the physician's order to ensure that no discrepancies exist.

2. Review the order to ensure that the oxygen concentration is prescribed.

3. If any part of the order is unfamiliar, question its accuracy.

B. *Review Chart.* Use the following procedure to review the patient's chart:

1. On the patient's chart, identify all pertinent data in the following areas:

   • History and physical
   • Admitting diagnosis
   • Progress notes
   • Blood gas analysis

2. Based on the patient data, identify the following:

   • Conditions that indicate the need for oxygen therapy
   • Potential hazards of oxygen for the patient

C. *Maintain Asepsis.* While performing the remainder of this procedure, you are expected to maintain aseptic conditions and follow universal precautions according to the procedure described in **SSE 1.2**. This includes washing your hands:

   • Before obtaining equipment
   • Following performance of *I. Monitor Patient*
   • Anytime during the procedure that contamination is suspected

D. *Obtain Equipment.* Collect the following equipment and supplies:

   • Oxygen hood
   • Oxygen flowmeter
   • Heated humidifier or low output heated nebulizer
   • Aerosol tubing
   • T-piece
   • Sterile water (or other prescribed solution)

E. *Assemble Equipment.* Prepare equipment for use as follows:

    1. Fill the humidifier to the mark with water.

    2. Connect the aerosol tubing between the humidifier outlet and the T-piece.

    3. Attach the oxygen flowmeter to the gas inlet of the humidifier.

F. *Test Equipment.* Test the equipment as follows:

    1. Test the humidifier or nebulizer according to the procedure described in **CPE 10.1**.

G. *Confirm Patient.* Ensure that the procedure is performed with the correct patient as follows:

    1. Match the information on the order with the following:

        • Room number
        • Name on the door or bed

    2. Resolve any discrepancies in the patient identification information by conferring with the nursing staff.

H. *Implement Procedure.* Perform the following tasks:

    1. Connect the oxygen flowmeter to the gas outlet.

    2. Turn on the flowmeter.

    3. Place the hood over the infant's head.

    4. Place the T-piece into the port in the back of the hood.

    5. Analyze the oxygen concentration by placing the analyzer probe close to the infant's face.

    6. Adjust the oxygen flow as necessary in order to obtain the desired oxygen concentration ordered by the physician.

I. *Monitor Patient.* Determine the patient's response to the therapy as follows:

    1. Determine the pulse rate. (Count for at least one minute.)

    2. Determine the respiratory rate. (Count for at least one minute.)

3. Observe respirations to identify any abnormalities in the breathing pattern.

4. Note any abnormalities in the patient's appearance or behavior.

J. *Record Results.* Document the therapy as follows:

1. Record the following data on the patient's chart:

   • Date
   • Time
   • FIO_2 delivered
   • Pulse rate
   • Respiratory rate
   • Abnormal patient characteristics

2. Sign the patient's chart (first initial and full last name).

K. *Report Observations.* Report the following information:

1. Report any significant adverse changes in the patient's condition to the nurse or physician whenever observed.

2. Following the procedure, report to the nurse or physician:

   • Any non-critical adverse reactions to the therapy
   • Other pertinent observations of the patient's condition

Evaluation of Oxygen Therapy for Infants

The following definitions are provided for use whenever the respective Clinical Procedures are evaluated. In order for performance of the procedures to be considered acceptable, all Essential Tasks are to be performed according to the accompanying Evaluation Criteria. Any deviation from the following task sequence or criteria must be approved in advance by the evaluator.

CPE 14.1 Infant Hood or Halo		
Performance	**Essential Tasks**	**Evaluation Criteria**
A. Check Order	See SSE 3.1	See SSE 3.1
B. Review Chart	See SSE 3.2	See SSE 3.2
C. Maintain Asepsis	See SSE 1.2	See SSE 1.2
D. Obtain Equipment	1. Obtains the following equipment and supplies: • Oxygen hood • Heated humidifier • Nebulizer • Aerosol tubing • T-piece • Sterile solution	a. Correct equipment obtained
E. Assemble Equipment	1. Prepares equipment for use as follows: • Fills humidifier • Assembles nebulizer, T-piece and halo	a. Sterile solution used b. Humidifier filled to mark c. Assembled according to **SOP**
F. Test Equipment	1. Tests for: • Functioning of equipment • Leaks in system	a. Tested according to **SOP** b. Leaks remedied c. Defective equipment replaced

CPE 14.1		
Infant Hood or Halo (continued)		
Performance	**Essential Tasks**	**Evaluation Criteria**
G. Confirm Patient	See SSE 3.3	See SSE 3.3
H. Implement Procedure	1. Administers therapy	a. Correct flow rate used. b. Correct oxygen concentration used
I. Monitor Patient	1. Determines: • Respiratory rate 2. Observes: • Respiratory pattern • Patient appearance	a. Counted for at least one (1) minute a. Any abnormalities identified
J. Record Results	See SSE 3.4	See SSE 3.4
K. Report Observations	See SSE 4.3	See SSE 4.3

Module 15.0

Ventilatory Assistance for Infants

This module pertains to the preparation and use of an infant mechanical ventilator for the administration of continuous positive airway pressure (CPAP) and continuous ventilation to infants. Procedures are outlined for the set-up, check and change-out of commonly used infant ventilators. CPAP is included in this module because the most common and the recommended method of administering CPAP is with an infant mechanical ventilator.

Objectives

Upon completion of this module, you will be able to:

1. List and explain the conditions that indicate the use of CPAP.

2. List and describe the potential hazards associated with CPAP.

3. List and explain the conditions that indicate the use of continuous mechanical ventilation.

4. List and describe the potential hazards associated with continuous mechanical ventilation.

5. Set-up, check and change-out an infant ventilator.

The most common neonatal disorder requiring ventilatory assistance is infant respiratory distress syndrome. This condition, also known as hyaline membrane disease, results from insufficient production of pulmonary surfactant by the immature lungs of the neonate. Pulmonary surfactant acts to prevent alveolar collapse on expiration. If insufficient surfactant is present, the neonate must exert an extremely high (40 to 80 cm H_2O) negative pressure in order to obtain an adequate tidal volume. Since surfactant usually develops between weeks 22 and 35 of the gestation period, hyaline membrane disease is most prevalent in premature infants.

The infant with hyaline membrane disease is usually symptomatic at birth or immediately after. The signs and symptoms presented usually include:

- Tachypnea
- Sternal and intercostal retractions
- Cyanosis
- Nasal flaring
- Expiratory grunting
- Hypoventilation
- Ground-glass appearance on chest x-ray

Alveolar collapse, associated with hyaline membrane disease, results in the occurrence of shunting and subsequent hypoxemia. In addition, pulmonary compliance is greatly reduced because alveolar collapse requires increased pressure to inflate the lungs. Consequently, the work of breathing necessary to maintain alveolar ventilation is greatly increased.

Many of the characteristics of continuous mechanical ventilators were described in **Module 13.0**. For use with neonates, the characteristics of a ventilator should include:

- Continuous flow
- Ability to deliver small tidal volumes
- Time cycling
- Wide range of respiratory rates
- Adjustable I:E ratios
- Rapid response time
- Pressure-limiting mechanism
- Control, IMV, and CPAP modes
- Humidification of inspired gas
- Adjustable FIO_2 concentrations

An infant ventilator is used whenever ventilatory assistance is required by the neonate. Adult ventilators are unable to deliver small tidal volumes accurately at the rapid rates required of a neonate. Since the tidal volume that can be delivered by an infant ventilator is limited, however, it is seldom used with infants weighing more than approximately 20 pounds.

Continuous Positive Airway Pressure

The safest and preferred method of providing CPAP to an infant is by means of an infant ventilator. CPAP can be provided via the endotracheal tube or nasal CPAP prongs. The infant ventilator provides a controlled flow rate and humidification, constant positive pressure at desired levels, a reliable oxygen source, and patient monitoring to indicate any changes in the pressure delivered. While in the CPAP mode, time cycling of the ventilator is bypassed and the infant initiates each breath. When administering CPAP, respiratory rate monitors must be employed to ensure that the infant's breathing rate is sufficient.

Indications

Whenever an adequate PaO_2 cannot be maintained by the delivery of supplemental oxygen at ambient pressure, more aggressive therapy is indicated. CPAP can be administered to infants who are breathing spontaneously and who are able to maintain a $PaCO_2$ less than 70 mm Hg and a pH greater than 7.25. By maintaining a constant positive pressure throughout the respiratory cycle, CPAP prevents alveolar collapse. For this reason, CPAP makes it possible to maintain an adequate PaO_2 without increasing FIO_2.

Hazards

The potential hazards of CPAP include all of the hazards associated with oxygen therapy. In addition, CPAP has the potential of causing hypotension, decreased cardiac output, and pneumothorax due to increased intrathoracic pressure.

Continuous Mechanical Ventilation

When other efforts to reduce the respiratory distress of a neonate have been unsuccessful, more intensive therapy may be required. Additional assistance can be provided by utilizing the time-cycling mechanism of the ventilator. This feature provides a fixed number of mandatory breaths to the infant. The continuous positive pressure required by hyaline membrane disease can be maintained by using the PEEP capability of the ventilator.

Indications

If the patient is apneic or is unable to maintain a $PaCO_2$ less than 70 mm Hg, mechanical ventilation is indicated. As with adults, continuous ventilation of an infant reduces the work of breathing and improves ventilatory efficiency by manipulating the respiratory pattern and airway pressures. Since the patient is subjected to considerable risk during mechanical ventilation, however, such therapy should only be administered when warranted by the potential benefits.

Hazards

The hazards associated with the use of adult mechanical ventilators were described in **Module 13.0**. Since the hazards accompanying the use of an infant ventilator are essentially the same, they will not be repeated.

Clinical Procedure 15.1
Infant Ventilator Set Up

The same equipment is used to administer both CPAP and continuous ventilation to neonates. However, CPAP may be administered via the endotracheal tube or nasal CPAP prongs. A seperate section will discuss nasal CPAP prongs.

Procedure for Performing an Infant Ventilator Set up

The following procedure is recommended for setting up a stand-by infant ventilator:

A. *Maintain Asepsis.* While performing the remainder of this procedure, you are expected to maintain aseptic conditions according to the procedure described in **SSE 1.2.** This includes washing your hands:

- Before obtaining equipment
- Following performance of *C. Assemble Equipment*
- Anytime during the procedure that contamination is suspected

B. *Obtain Equipment.* Collect the following equipment and supplies:

- Ventilator
- Infant circuit
- Humidifier system
- Test lung
- Oxygen analyzer
- Stethoscope

C. *Assemble Equipment.* Prepare the equipment for use as follows:

1. Attach ventilator circuit to ventilator at humidifier outlet and ventilator inlet.

2. Connect humidifier to ventilator outlet. (Do not fill humidifier or break seal on water.)

3. Attach test lung.

4. Tighten all fittings.

D. ***Test Equipment.*** Test the ventilator as follows:

1. Connect the ventilator to the air and oxygen gas outlets.

2. If the gas oxygen blender alarm sounds, check the gas supply tubing to assure:

   • Tubings are not kinked or obstructed.
   • Tubings are properly connected to the gas outlets.
   • Water condensate is not obstructing the air supply.

3. If the oxygen blender alarm still sounds, check the inlet pressure gauge to assure:

   • Adequate pressure from both gas sources.
   • Pressure difference does not exceed 20 psi.

4. Adjust the gas supplies as needed.

5. If the gas outlet pressures are correct and no obstructions to gas flow are noted, yet the alarm is still sounding:

   • Label the blender or ventilator as "defective" and replace it.
   • Reassemble and retest the new equipment.

6. Calibrate the oxygen analyzer and place it in line with the circuit between the ventilator outlet and humidifier.

7. Check oxygen percentage delivered by the machine at 40%. If analyzer does not read 40% $\pm$ 3 within two minutes label it as defective.

8. Check the ventalator according to specific manufacturer guidelines.

9. Cover and store in a convenient location.

Clinical Procedure 15.2
Infant Ventilator Check

This section of the module presents the procedures used to perform a check on an infant ventilator. The ventilator check procedures are essentially the same regardless of whether the patient is receiving CPAP or continuous ventilation. The minor differences which do exist are indicated in the following procedures by the use of asterisks.

Procedure for Performing an Infant Ventilator Check

It is recommended that an infant ventilator check be performed according to the following procedure:

A. *Maintain Asepsis.* While performing the remainder of this procedure, you are expected to maintain aseptic conditions and observe universal precautions according to the procedure described in **SSE 1.2**. This includes washing your hands:

- Before obtaining equipment
- Following performance of *F. Report Observations*
- Anytime during the procedure that contamination is suspected

B. *Obtain Equipment.* Collect the following equipment and supplies:

- Stethoscope
- Oxygen analyzer
- Suction equipment

C. *Confirm Patient.* Ensure that the procedure is performed with the correct patient as follows:

1. Match the information on the order with the following:

- Room number
- Name on the door or bed

2. Resolve any discrepancies in the patient identification information by conferring with the nursing staff.

D. **Implement Procedure.** Perform the following tasks:

1. *Assess Appearance.* Assess the infant's appearance regarding color, state of consciousness and agitation and record the results.

2. *Empty Condensate.* Empty condensate from the ventilator tubing, moving water away from the patient into the appropriate reservoir (i.e., wastebasket, *not* the humidifier).

3. *Wash Hands.* Wash your hands according to the procedure described in **SSE 1.1**.

4. *Auscultate Chest.* Auscultate the patient's chest according to the procedure described in **SSE 2.2**. If rales are audible, suction the patient according to the procedure described in **APE 8.1**.

5. *Check Pulse.* Count for at least one minute and record the results.

6. *Check Respiratory Rate.* If in the IPPV/IMV mode, compare the respiratory rate ordered by the physician with the patient's actual respiratory rate and record the results.

7. *Check Airway Pressure.* If the desired proximal airway pressure is not generated, either adjust the flow rate or the pressure limit control and record the results.

8. *Check I:E Ratio.* Check the I:E ratio time and adjust as necessary to obtain the ratio ordered by the physician and record the results.

9. *Analyze FIO_2.* If necessary, adjust the inspired oxygen concentration in order to maintain the FIO_2 ordered by the physician and record the results.

10. *Check PEEP or CPAP.* Adjust the controls as necessary in order to obtain the PEEP or CPAP mode ordered by the physician and record the results.

11. *Check Temperature.* Check the temperature of the inspired gas and, if necessary, adjust the heater in order to maintain $98 \pm 2°F$ and record the results.

12. *Check Humidifier.* Check the fluid level of the humidifier and add the prescribed solution as needed.

13. *Check Alarms.* Check the operation of all alarms on or adapted to the ventilator to assure that all lights, fuses and/or batteries are functioning properly.

E. **Record Results.** Document the ventilator check as follows:

1. Record:

   - Breath sounds
   - Sputum volume, color, and consistency
   - Other pertinent information

2. Make certain that all of the following results obtained in Steps 1 through 13 above were recorded clearly:

   - Pulse rate
   - Respiratory rate(s)
   - Proximal airway pressure
   - I:E ratio*
   - FIO_2
   - Temperature
   - PEEP or CPAP
   - Other applicable parameters
     (*This is not applicable when administering CPAP.)

F. **Report Observations.** Report the following information:

1. Report any significant adverse changes in the patient's condition to the nurse or physician whenever observed.

2. Following the procedure, report to the nurse or physician:

   - Any non-critical adverse reactions to the therapy
   - Other pertinent observations of the patient's condition

Clinical Procedure 15.3
Infant Ventilator Change-Out

The same equipment is used to administer both CPAP and continuous ventilation to neonates. This section of the module presents the procedures used to change-out infant ventilators. Depending on the type of equipment available, follow the steps as applicable to change-out the particular infant ventilator that you are using. When replacing continuous ventilation equipment, always exercise due caution to ensure adequate ventilation of the infant at all times.

Procedure for Performing an Infant Ventilator Change-Out

Whenever it is necessary to perform a ventilator change-out, the following general procedure is recommended:

A. *Maintain Asepsis.* While performing the remainder of this procedure, you are expected to maintain aseptic conditions and follow universal precautions according to the procedure described in **SSE 1.2**. This includes washing your hands:

  • Before obtaining equipment
  • Following performance of **E. Report Observations**
  • Anytime during the procedure that contamination is suspected

B. *Obtain Equipment.* Collect the following equipment and supplies:

  • Ventilator
  • Infant circuit
  • Humidifier system
  • Oxygen analyzer
  • Stethoscope
  • Resuscitation bag and mask

C. *Confirm Patient.* Ensure that the procedure is performed with the correct patient as follows:

  1. Match the information on the order with the following:

    • Room number
    • Name on the door or bed

2. Resolve any discrepancies in the patient identification information by conferring with the nursing staff.

D.   *Implement Procedure.* Perform the following tasks:

1. Assemble ventilator circuit and attach to humidifier outlet.

2. *Perform Ventilator Check.* Perform a ventilator check according to the procedure described in **CPE 15.2**.

3. *Breathe Patient.* In preparation for disconnection from the ventilator, manually breathe the patient by compressing the manual resuscitation bag.

4. *Change Circuit.* Replace with the clean circuit as follows:

   • Disconnect the used circuit form the ventilator outlet and replace it with the clean circuit.
   • Replace the oxygen analyzer in the circuit.
   • Assemble the ventilator circuit and attach to the humidifier outlet.

5. *Breathe Patient.* Repeat Step 3 above.

6. *Fill Nebulizer.* Fill the nebulizer with the prescribed solution (as applicable).

7. *Perform Ventilator Check.* Perform a ventilator check according to the procedure described in **CPE 15.2**.

E.   *Report Observations.* Report the following information:

1. Report any significant adverse changes in the patient's condition to the nurse or physician whenever observed.

2. Following the procedure, report to the nurse or physician:

   • Any non-critical adverse reactions to the therapy
   • Other pertinent observations of the patient's condition

Evaluation of Ventilatory Assistance for Infants

The following definitions are provided for use whenever the respective Clinical Procedures are evaluated. In order for performance of the procedures to be considered acceptable, all Essential Tasks are to be performed according to the accompanying Evaluation Criteria. Any deviation from the following task sequence or criteria must be approved by the evaluator.

CPE 15.1 Ventilator Set Up		
Performance	**Essential Tasks**	**Evaluation Criteria**
A. Maintain Asepsis	See **SSE 1.2**	See **SSE 1.2**
B. Obtain Equipment	1. Obtains the following equipment and supplies: • Ventilator • Infant circuit • Humidifier system • Test lung • Oxygen analyzer • Stethoscope	a. Correct equipment obtained
C. Assemble Equipment	1. Prepares equipment as follows: • Attaches ventilator circuit to humidifier circuit • Connects humidifier to ventilator outlet • Attaches test lung • Tightens all fittings	a. Assembled according to **SOP**
D. Test Equipment	1. Tests for: • Oxygen concentration • Functioning of equipment • Leaks in system	a. Tested according to **SOP** b. Defective equipment replaced c. Defective equipment identified d. Leaks remedied

CPE 15.2 Ventilator Check		
Performance	**Essential Tasks**	**Evaluation Criteria**
A. Maintain Asepsis	See **SSE 1.2**	See **SSE 1.2**
B. Obtain Equipment	1. Obtains the following equipment and supplies: • Stethoscope • Oxygen analyzer • Suction equipment	a. Correct equipment obtained
C. Confirm Patient	See **SSE 3.3**	See **SSE 3.3**
D. Implement Procedure	1. Determines the following patient characteristics: • Color • State of consciousness • Agitation	a. Assessed correctly
	2. Empties condensate	a. Emptied away from patient b. Emptied into appropriate reservoir (not humidifier)
	3. Washes hands	a. Performed according to **SSE 1.1**
	4. Auscultates chest	a. Performed according to **SSE 2.2**
	5. Checks pulse	a. Counted for at least one (1) minute b. Results recorded
	6. Checks respiratory rate.	a. Counted for at least one (1) minute b. Actual value compared with ordered value c. Results recorded
	7. Checks airway pressure	a. Adjusted when necessary b. Results recorded

CPE 15.2
Ventilator Checks (continued)

Performance	Essential Tasks	Evaluation CRiteria
D. Implement Procedure (continued)	8. Checks inspiratory rate	a. Adjusted when necessary
	9. Checks expiratory time	a. Adjusted when necessary
	10. Analyzes FIO_2	a. FIO_2 administered compared with order b. FIO_2 adjusted when necessary to compare with other c. Results recorded
	11. Checks PEEP or CPAP	a. Adjusted when necessary b. Results recorded
	12. Checks nebulizer	a. Fluid level checked b. Sterile solution added if necessary
	13. Checks alarms	a. Fuses and/or batteries functioned properly
E. Record Results	1. Records the following data: • Breath sounds • Sputum volume • Sputum color • Sputum consistency • Other pertinent information	a. Only factual information recorded b. No important details omitted c. No irrelevant data recorded d. All information accurate e. All errors properly corrected
	2. Assures recording of the following: • Temperature • Pulse rate • Respiratory rate(s) • Proximal airway pressure • I:E ratio • FIO_2 • PEEP or CPAP • Other applicable parameters	a. Only factual information recorded b. No important details omitted c. No irrelevant data recorded d. All information accurate e. All errors properly corrected
F. Report Observations	See SSE 4.3	See SSE 4.3

CPE 15.3 Ventilator Change-Out		
Performance	**Essential Tasks**	**Evaluation Criteria**
A. Maintain Asepsis	See SSE 1.2	See SSE 1.2
B. Obtain Equipment	1. Obtains the following equipment and supplies: • Circuit • Humidifier system • Oxygen analyzer • Stethoscope • Resuscitation bag and mask	a. Correct equipment obtained
C. Confirm Patient	See SSE 3.3	See SSE 3.3
D. Implement Procedure	1. Assembles equipment	a. Circuit assembled according to **SOP**
	2. Performs ventilator check	a. Performed according to **CPE 15.2**
	3. Breathes patient	a. Manual deep breaths provided
	4. Changes circuit	a. Nebulizer replaced b. Circuit replaced
	5. Breathes patient	a. Manual deep breaths provided
	6. Fills nebulizer	a. Nebulizer filled to mark b. Sterile solution added
	7. Breathes patient	a. Manual deep breaths provided
	8. Performs ventilator check	a. Performed according to **CPE 15.2**
E. Report Observations	See SSE 4.3	See SSE 4.3

Section Four
Evaluation Procedures

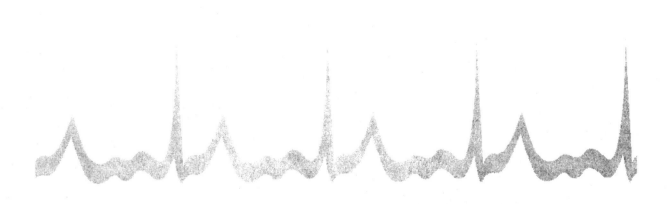

Proficiency Evaluation Process

Evaluation Procedures

It is important that you understand the procedures for performing a clinical evaluation. The information collected should be as complete and accurate as possible. When used correctly, the instruments are designed to facilitate objectivity on the part of the evaluator. The procedures for conducting a clinical evaluation are as follows:

Before the Evaluation

1. Thoroughly familiarize yourself with the evaluation instruments. By reducing your reliance on the "Essential Task" and "Evaluation Criteria" definitions, you can direct more attention to observing the student's performance during the evaluation session.

2. Meet with the student at the scheduled time to discuss the procedures to be followed and to answer any questions.

3. Review the respiratory care order and the patient's chart to become familiar with any pertinent conditions. Since the student will discuss the chart data and their implications for the therapy with you, it may be good to make notes in advance.

4. Advise the student that, except for any agreed upon deviations, the procedure is to be performed exactly as described in the manual. Any deviations should be noted on the Proficiency Evaluation Form.

5. Encourage the student to perform the procedure and interact with the patient in the same manner that would be followed if you were not present. The only exceptions are as follows:

   a. During order confirmation and chart review, the data and any conclusions drawn from the data should be reviewed with you.

   b. The results of any nonobservable activities should be expressed verbally (e.g., respiratory rate or heart rate).

6. Advise the student that you are only an observer and that any assistance which must be given (either with or without a request from the student) may result in an unacceptable evaluation.

7. Attempt to reduce any apparent fears and anxieties that the student may have regarding the evaluation session.

8. Record all identification information on the top of the Proficiency Evaluation Form.

During the Evaluation

9. Inform the student of the procedure to be evaluated, the patient selected and the patient's location. (From this point on, you are an observer. Any further information given to the student should pertain only to the evaluation process, not to the procedure being performed.)

10. Explain to the student that any nonobservable tasks are to be described verbally. (During chart review, it may be necessary to quiz the student orally. If so, be careful not to provide information which may assist the student in performing this step.)

11. Accompany the student during the entire procedure (e.g., to where the chart is kept, to the equipment storage area, to the patient's room, etc.).

12. Explain the purpose of your presence to the patient. (Ordinarily this should be done by the student.)

13. Find a position where you can observe each step of the procedure unobtrusively.

14. As the student completes each step of the procedure, record the performance on the Proficiency Evaluation Form. (Follow the data recording procedures provided in the next section of these instructions.)

15. Ask any questions necessary to clarify your observations. (Questions should be asked at a time and in a manner that will minimize distracting the student and the patient. If possible, delay questions until the procedure is completed.)

16. While the procedure is being performed, provide no assistance of any kind to the student. (The only exception is if you happen to observe something which is endangering the patient.)

17. If a student makes numerous errors or even one critical error which may endanger the patient, terminate the evaluation and assist with completion of the procedure.

18. Following completion of the procedure, record any additional comments or explanatory remarks in the space provided on the Proficiency Evaluation Form.

19. Repeat each step in the evaluation process with each procedure to be evaluated.

Following the Evaluation

20. Review and discuss the evaluation results for each procedure with the student.

21. Get the student's signature on each Proficiency Evaluation Form (preferably immediately following the discussion of each procedure).

22. If any procedures were performed in an unacceptable manner, explain to the student that another evaluation session will have to be scheduled.

23. If any procedures were performed in an unacceptable manner, you are encouraged to make two copies of the Proficiency Evaluation Form for the procedure. One copy should be given to the student and the other retained by yourself.

24. Go over the Proficiency Evaluation Forms one more time to make certain that all are complete and contain your signature.

25. Mail the completed Proficiency Evaluation Forms to CCHS.

Data Recording Procedures

All data is recorded on the Proficiency Evaluation Forms. A specific form is provided for each procedure to be evaluated. The Evaluation Instruments define and describe the correct method of performing the procedures. You should use the instruments to determine whether the student performs the procedures in an unacceptable manner, but not for recording evaluation results. The instruments are yours to keep and to use when conducting evaluations in the future.

Note: The example presents a variety of potential student errors. It is unlikely that a single student would make all these errors. In fact, students are expected to perform the procedure without error.

The following procedures are used to complete the Proficiency Evaluation Forms. An example of a completed form is provided for reference.

1. Record the information requested on top of the form.

2. When evaluation of a procedure begins, record the time in the space provided.

3. As each step in the procedure is performed, circle the letter indicating the correct score as follows:

   a. If all Essential Tasks are performed according to the Evaluation Criteria (see Evaluation Instruments), circle "A" for acceptable.

   b. If any Essential Tasks are omitted or performed incorrectly as defined by the Evaluation Criteria, circle "U" for unacceptable.

   c. If any Performance Step is omitted entirely or was unobservable, circle "N" for not evaluated.

4. In most instances, the Performance Steps and Essential Tasks must be performed in the sequence given. Although certain minor deviations may be acceptable, others may

constitute "incorrect procedure." If a procedure is performed in an order which you consider a critical deviation from the sequence given, score the step "U."

5. For any "U" or "N" scores, write a brief comment in the space provided as follows:

    a. If an Essential Task was omitted, write the number of the task in the comment column.

    b. If an Evaluation Criterion was violated for an Essential Task, write the number of the task and the letter of the criterion in the comment column.

    c. Briefly explain any "N" score.

    d. Add other explanatory comments which pertain to a particular Performance Step as needed.

6. When the procedure is completed, record the time in the space provided.

7. Determine and record the results of the evaluation at the top of the form. An acceptable ("A") result indicates that the procedure was performed without error (no scores of "U"). Ordinarily, a score of "N" on one of the Performance Steps will result in an unacceptable ("U") evaluation.

8. Record any additional comments or explanatory remarks in the space provided at the bottom of the form.

9. Compute the time in minutes required for performing the procedure and record it in the space provided.

10. Sign the Proficiency Evaluation Form.

11. Review the results of the evaluation with the student and obtain the student's signature.

Proficiency Evaluation Form

Location __MEMORIAL HOSPITAL__ Student __MICHAEL RODGERS__

Date __3/18/93__   Evaluation Results   A (U)

Unusual Patient Characteristics __NONE__

Time: Start __9:35 a.m.__ Stop __9:50 a.m.__ Total __15__ (minutes)

Performance	Results	Comments
A. Check Order	(A) U N	
B. Review Chart	A (U) N	2. (BLOOD GAS DATA NOT REVIEWED)
C. Maintain Asepsis	A (U) N	1.b. (HANDS NOT WASHED AFTER)
D. Obtain Equipment	(A) U N	
E. Assemble Equipment	(A) U N	
F. Test Equipment	(A) U N	
G. Confirm Patient	A U (N)	ALREADY KNEW PATIENT
H. Inform Patient	(A) U N	
I. Implement Procedure	A (U) N	1.b. (SIGN NOT POSTED IN ROOM) 2.c. (ASSISTANCE NEEDED)
J. Monitor Patient	(A) U N	
K. Conclude Procedure	(A) U N	
L. Record Results	A U (N)	EVALUATION TERMINATED
M. Report Observations	A U (N)	

Additional Comments: STUDENT WAS OBVIOUSLY UNPREPARED, IT WAS NEC-ESSARY TO PROVIDE HELP WITH RESERVOIR BAG TO ENSURE PROPER FIO_2 DELIVERY. STUDENT COMPLETED STEPS J. & K. — THEN EVALUATION SESSION WAS TERMINATED. EVALUATION WILL HAVE TO BE RESCHEDULED.

Signatures:

Student __Michael Rodgers__   Evaluator __Lori Wieronski__

Evaluation of Oxygen Administration Procedures

The following definitions are provided for use whenever oxygen administration procedures are evaluated. In order for performance of the procedure to be considered acceptable, all Essential Tasks are to be performed according to the accompanying Evaluation Criteria. Any deviation from the following task sequence or criteria must be approved by the evaluator.

EXAMPLE

CPE 9.1 Oxygen Therapy		
Performance	**Essential Tasks**	**Evaluation Criteria**
A. Check Order	See **SSE 3.1**	See **SSE 3.1**
B. Review Chart	See **SSE 3.2** *2. DID NOT IDENTIFY + DISCUSS BLOOD GAS DATA*	See **SSE 3.2**
C. Maintain Asepsis	See **SSE 1.2**	See **SSE 1.2** *1.b DID NOT WASH HANDS AFTER PROCEDURE*
D. Obtain Equipment	1. Obtains the following equipment and supplies: • Oxygen flowmeter • Humidifier • Sterile water • Oxygen supply tubing • Prescribed delivery device • "No Smoking" signs	a. Correct equipment obtained
E. Assemble Equipment	1. Prepares equipment as follows: • Fills humidifier • Assembles humidifier, tubing, tubing, and flowmeter	a. Sterile water used b. Humidifier filled c. Assembled according to order and **SOP**
F. Test Equipment	1. Tests for: • Functioning of alarm • Leaks in system	a. Tested according to **SOP** b. Leaks remedied c. Defective equipment replaced
G. Confirm Patient	See **SSE 3.3**	See **SSE 3.3** *DID NOT PERFORM ALL STEPS — ALREADY KNEW PATIENT*

CPE 9.1
Oxygen Therapy (continued)

Performance	Essential Tasks	Evaluation Criteria
H. Inform Patient	See SSE 4.1	See SSE 4.1 *OK – SHOULD USE LESS TECHNICAL LANGUAGE*
I. Implement Procedure	1. Posts "No Smoking" signs	a. Posted on the door (b.) Posted above bed or in other suitable location *NOT DONE*
	2. Administers therapy	a. Correct flow rate used b. Delivery device attached correctly (c.) If bag used, maintained at least 1/3 full *ASSISTANCE PROVIDED*
J. Monitor Patient	1. Determines: • Pulse rate • Respiratory rate	a. Counted for at least one (1) minute
	2. Observes: • Respiratory pattern • Patient appearance	a. Any abnormalities identified
K. Conclude Procedure	1. Replaces call bell and bedside table	a. Placed within patient's reach
	2. Tends to patient needs	a. Comfortable position assured b. Patient asked regarding other needs c. Patient questions answered effectively – *NONE ASKED BY PT.*
L. Record Results	See SSE 3.4 *RR NOT RECORDED – PROCEDURE TERMINATED*	See SSE 3.4
M. Report Observations	See SSE 4.3	See SSE 4.3

Proficiency Evaluation Form

Location _____ Student _____

Date _____ Evaluation Results | A   U |

Unusual Patient Characteristics _____

Time: Start _____ Stop _____ Total _____ (minutes)

Performance	Results	Comments
A. Clean Equipment	A U N	
B. Immerse Equipment	A U N	
C. Rinse Items	A U N	
D. Dry Items	A U N	
E. Assemble Equipment	A U N	
F. Package Equipment	A U N	
G. Store Equipment	A U N	

Additional Comments:

Signatures:

Student _____ Evaluator _____

Proficiency Evaluation Form

Location _____ Student _____

Date _____ Evaluation Results | A   U |

Unusual Patient Characteristics _____

Time: Start _____ Stop _____ Total _____ (minutes)

Performance	Results	Comments
A. Clean Equipment	A U N	
B. Immerse Equipment	A U N	
C. Dry Items	A U N	
D. Assemble Equipment	A U N	
E. Package Equipment	A U N	
F. Store Equipment	A U N	

Additional Comments:

Signatures:

Student _____ Evaluator _____

Proficiency Evaluation Form

Location _____ Student _____

Date _____ Evaluation Results | A   U |

Unusual Patient Characteristics _____

Time: Start _____ Stop _____ Total _____ (minutes)

Performance	Results	Comments
A. Clean Equipment	A U N	
B. Assemble Equipment	A U N	
C. Package Equipment	A U N	
D. Label Packages	A U N	
E. Position Packages	A U N	
F. Operate Autoclave	A U N	
G. Store Equipment	A U N	

Additional Comments:

Signatures:

Student _____ Evaluator _____

Proficiency Evaluation Form

Location _____ Student _____

Date _____ Evaluation Results [A   U]

Unusual Patient Characteristics _____

Time: Start _____ Stop _____ Total _____ (minutes)

Performance	Results	Comments
A. Clean Equipment	A U N	
B. Assemble Equipment	A U N	
C. Package Equipment	A U N	
D. Label Packages	A U N	
E. Position Packages	A U N	
F. Operate Sterilizer	A U N	
G. Aerate Equipment	A U N	
H. Store Equipment	A U N	

Additional Comments:

Signatures:

Student _____ Evaluator _____

Proficiency Evaluation Form

Location _____ Student _____

Date _____ Evaluation Results | A   U |

Unusual Patient Characteristics _____

Time: Start _____ Stop _____ Total _____ (minutes)

Performance	Results	Comments
A. Maintain Asepsis	A U N	
B. Prepare Equipment	A U N	
C. Confirm Patient	A U N	
D. Inform Patient	A U N	
E. Demonstrate FVC, V_T and $\dot{V}_E$ Procedures	A U N	
F. Implement FVC, V_T and $\dot{V}_E$ Procedures	A U N	
G. Demonstrate MIP Procedures	A U N	
H. Implement MIP Procedures	A U N	
I. Conclude Procedure	A U N	
J. Record Results	A U N	
K. Report Observations	A U N	

Additional Comments:

Signatures:

Student _____ Evaluator _____

Proficiency Evaluation Form

Location _____   Student _____

Date _____   Evaluation Results | A   U |

Unusual Patient Characteristics _____

Time: Start _____   Stop _____   Total _____ (minutes)

Performance	Results	Comments
A. Check Order	A U N	
B. Assure Stabilization	A U N	
C. Maintain Asepsis	A U N	
D. Obtain Equipment	A U N	
E. Assemble Equipment	A U N	
F. Confirm Patient	A U N	
G. Inform Patient	A U N	
H. Perform Allen Test	A U N	
I. Implement Procedure	A U N	
J. Monitor Patient	A U N	
K. Record Data	A U N	
L. Conclude Procedure	A U N	
J. Monitor Patient	A U N	
M. Report Observations	A U N	
N. Dispense Sample	A U N	

Additional Comments:

Signatures:

Student _____   Evaluator _____

Proficiency Evaluation Form

Location _____ Student _____

Date _____ Evaluation Results | A   U |

Unusual Patient Characteristics _____

Time: Start _____ Stop _____ Total _____ (minutes)

Performance	Results	Comments
A. Check Order	A U N	
B. Assure Stabilization	A U N	
C. Maintain Asepsis	A U N	
D. Obtain Equipment	A U N	
E. Assemble Equipment	A U N	
F. Confirm Patient	A U N	
G. Inform Patient	A U N	
H. Assess Perfusion to Site	A U N	
I. Implement Procedure	A U N	
J. Monitor Patient	A U N	
K. Record Data	A U N	
L. Conclude Procedure	A U N	
M. Report Observations	A U N	

Additional Comments:

Signatures:

Student _____ Evaluator _____

Proficiency Evaluation Form

Location _____ Student _____

Date _____ Evaluation Results | A   U |

Unusual Patient Characteristics _____

Time: Start _____ Stop _____ Total _____ (minutes)

Performance	Results	Comments
A. Check Order	A U N	
B. Maintain Asepsis	A U N	
C. Obtain Equipment	A U N	
D. Assemble Equipment	A U N	
E. Confirm Patient	A U N	
F. Inform Patient	A U N	
G. Implement Patient	A U N	
H. Monitor Patient	A U N	
I. Record Data	A U N	
J. Conclude Procedure	A U N	
K. Report Observations	A U N	

Additional Comments:

Signatures:

Student _____ Evaluator _____

Proficiency Evaluation Form

Location _____   Student _____

Date _____   Evaluation Results | A   U |

Unusual Patient Characteristics _____

Time: Start _____ Stop _____ Total _____ (minutes)

Performance	Results	Comments
A. Check Order	A U N	
B. Maintain Asepsis	A U N	
C. Obtain Equipment	A U N	
D. Assemble Equipment	A U N	
E. Confirm Patient	A U N	
F. Inform Patient	A U N	
G. Implement Procedure	A U N	
H. Monitor Patient	A U N	
I. Record Data	A U N	
J. Conclude Procedure	A U N	
K. Report Observations	A U N	

Additional Comments:

Signatures:

Student _____   Evaluator _____

Proficiency Evaluation Form

Location _____ Student _____

Date _____ Evaluation Results | A   U |

Unusual Patient Characteristics _____

Time: Start _____ Stop _____ Total _____ (minutes)

Performance	Results	Comments
A. Demonstrate Procedure	A U N	
B. Position Patient	A U N	
C. Coach Patient	A U N	
D. Complete Procedure	A U N	

Additional Comments:

Signatures:

Student _____ Evaluator _____

Proficiency Evaluation Form

Location _____ Student _____

Date _____ Evaluation Results | A   U |

Unusual Patient Characteristics _____

Time: Start _____ Stop _____ Total _____ (minutes)

Performance	Results	Comments
A. Demonstrate Procedure	A U N	
B. Coach Patient	A U N	
C. Complete Procedure	A U N	

Additional Comments:

Signatures:

Student _____ Evaluator _____

Proficiency Evaluation Form

Location _____ Student _____

Date _____ Evaluation Results | A   U |

Unusual Patient Characteristics _____

Time: Start _____ Stop _____ Total _____ (minutes)

Performance	Results	Comments
A. Demonstrate Procedure	A U N	
B. Position Patient	A U N	
C. Coach Patient	A U N	
D. Complete Procedure	A U N	

Additional Comments:

Signatures:

Student _____ Evaluator _____

Proficiency Evaluation Form

Location _____ Student _____

Date _____ Evaluation Results | A | U |

Unusual Patient Characteristics _____

Time: Start _____ Stop _____ Total _____ (minutes)

Performance	Results	Comments
A. Maintain Asepsis	A U N	
B. Obtain Equipment	A U N	
C. Assemble Equipment	A U N	
D. Test Equipment	A U N	
E. Confirm Patient	A U N	
F. Inform Patient	A U N	
G. Implement Procedure	A U N	
H. Conclude Procedure	A U N	
I. Record Results	A U N	
J. Report Observations	A U N	

Additional Comments:

Signatures:

Student _____ Evaluator _____

Proficiency Evaluation Form

Location _____   Student _____

Date _____   Evaluation Results | A   U |

Unusual Patient Characteristics _____

Time: Start _____ Stop _____ Total _____ (minutes)

Performance	Results	Comments
A. Maintain Asepsis	A U N	
B. Obtain Equipment	A U N	
C. Confirm Patient	A U N	
D. Inform Patient	A U N	
E. Implement Procedure	A U N	
F. Conclude Procedure	A U N	
G. Record Results	A U N	
H. Report Observations	A U N	

Additional Comments:

Signatures:

Student _____   Evaluator _____

Proficiency Evaluation Form

Location _____ Student _____

Date _____ Evaluation Results | A   U |

Unusual Patient Characteristics _____

Time: Start _____ Stop _____ Total _____ (minutes)

Performance	Results	Comments
A. Check Order	A U N	
B. Review Chart	A U N	
C. Maintain Asepsis	A U N	
D. Obtain Equipment	A U N	
E. Assemble Equipment	A U N	
F. Test Equipment	A U N	
G. Confirm Patient	A U N	
H. Inform Patient	A U N	
I. Implement Procedure	A U N	
J. Monitor Patient	A U N	
K. Conclude Procedure	A U N	
L. Report Observations	A U N	

Additional Comments:

Signatures:

Student _____ Evaluator _____

Proficiency Evaluation Form

Location _____ Student _____

Date _____ Evaluation Results | A   U |

Unusual Patient Characteristics _____

Time: Start _____ Stop _____ Total _____ (minutes)

Performance	Results	Comments
A. Check Order	A U N	
B. Maintain Aespsis	A U N	
C. Obtain Equipment	A U N	
D. Confirm Patient	A U N	
E. Inform Patient	A U N	
F. Implement Procedure	A U N	
G. Conclude Procedure	A U N	
H. Record Results	A U N	
I. Report Observations	A U N	

Additional Comments:

Signatures:

Student _____ Evaluator _____

Proficiency Evaluation Form

Location _____   Student _____

Date _____   Evaluation Results | A   U |

Unusual Patient Characteristics _____

Time: Start _____   Stop _____   Total _____ (minutes)

Performance	Results	Comments
A. Check Order	A U N	
B. Maintain Aespsis	A U N	
C. Obtain Equipment	A U N	
D. Confirm Patient	A U N	
E. Inform Patient	A U N	
F. Implement Procedure	A U N	
G. Conclude Procedure	A U N	
H. Record Results	A U N	
I. Report Observations	A U N	

Additional Comments:

Signatures:

Student _____   Evaluator _____

Proficiency Evaluation Form

Location _____ Student _____

Date _____ Evaluation Results [A   U]

Unusual Patient Characteristics _____

Time: Start _____ Stop _____ Total _____ (minutes)

Performance	Results	Comments
A. Check Order	A U N	
B. Review Chart	A U N	
C. Maintain Asepsis	A U N	
D. Obtain Equipment	A U N	
E. Assemble Equipment	A U N	
F. Test Equipment	A U N	
G. Confirm Patient	A U N	
H. Inform Patient	A U N	
I. Implement Procedure	A U N	
J. Monitor Patient	A U N	
K. Conclude Procedure	A U N	
L. Record Results	A U N	
M. Report Observations	A U N	

Additional Comments:

Signatures:

Student _____ Evaluator _____

Proficiency Evaluation Form

Location _____ Student _____

Date _____ Evaluation Results | A   U |

Unusual Patient Characteristics _____

Time: Start _____ Stop _____ Total _____ (minutes)

Performance	Results	Comments
A. Check Order	A U N	
B. Review Chart	A U N	
C. Maintain Asepsis	A U N	
D. Obtain Equipment	A U N	
E. Assemble Equipment	A U N	
F. Test Equipment	A U N	
G. Confirm Patient	A U N	
H. Inform Patient	A U N	
I. Implement Procedure	A U N	
J. Monitor Patient	A U N	
K. Conclude Procedure	A U N	
L. Record Results	A U N	
M. Report Observations	A U N	

Additional Comments:

Signatures:

Student _____ Evaluator _____

Proficiency Evaluation Form

Location _____   Student _____

Date _____   Evaluation Results | A   U |

Unusual Patient Characteristics _____

Time: Start _____ Stop _____ Total _____ (minutes)

Performance	Results	Comments
A. Check Order	A U N	
B. Review Chart	A U N	
C. Maintain Asepsis	A U N	
D. Obtain Equipment	A U N	
E. Assemble Equipment	A U N	
F. Test Equipment	A U N	
G. Confirm Patient	A U N	
H. Inform Patient	A U N	
I. Ensure Hygiene	A U N	
J. Implement Procedure	A U N	
K. Monitor Patient	A U N	
L. Coach Coughing	A U N	
M. Collect Sputum	A U N	
N. Conclude Procedure	A U N	
O. Record Results	A U N	
P. Report Observations	A U N	
Q. Dispense Specimen	A U N	

Additional Comments:

Signatures:

Student _____   Evaluator _____

Proficiency Evaluation Form

Location _____ Student _____

Date _____ Evaluation Results [A   U]

Unusual Patient Characteristics _____

Time: Start _____ Stop _____ Total _____ (minutes)

Performance	Results	Comments
A. Check Order	A U N	
B. Review Chart	A U N	
C. Maintain Asepsis	A U N	
D. Obtain Equipment	A U N	
E. Assemble Equipment	A U N	
F. Test Equipment	A U N	
G. Confirm Patient	A U N	
H. Inform Patient	A U N	
I. Implement Procedure	A U N	
J. Monitor Patient	A U N	
K. Conclude Procedure	A U N	
L. Record Results	A U N	
M. Report Observations	A U N	

Additional Comments:

Signatures:

Student _____ Evaluator _____

Proficiency Evaluation Form

Location _____ Student _____

Date _____ Evaluation Results | A   U |

Unusual Patient Characteristics _____

Time: Start _____ Stop _____ Total _____ (minutes)

Performance	Results	Comments
A. Check Order	A U N	
B. Review Chart	A U N	
C. Maintain Asepsis	A U N	
D. Obtain Equipment	A U N	
E. Assemble Equipment	A U N	
F. Confirm Patient	A U N	
G. Inform Patient	A U N	
H. Implement Procedure	A U N	
I. Monitor Patient	A U N	
J. Conclude Procedure	A U N	
K. Record Results	A U N	
L. Report Observations	A U N	

Additional Comments:

Signatures:

Student _____ Evaluator _____

Proficiency Evaluation Form

Location _____ Student _____

Date _____ Evaluation Results | A   U |

Unusual Patient Characteristics _____

Time: Start _____ Stop _____ Total _____ (minutes)

Performance	Results	Comments
A. Check Order	A U N	
B. Review Chart	A U N	
C. Maintain Asepsis	A U N	
D. Obtain Equipment	A U N	
E. Assemble Equipment	A U N	
F. Test Equipment	A U N	
G. Confirm Patient	A U N	
H. Inform Patient	A U N	
I. Implement Procedure	A U N	
J. Monitor Patient	A U N	
K. Conclude Procedure	A U N	
L. Record Results	A U N	
M. Report Observations	A U N	

Additional Comments:

Signatures:

Student _____ Evaluator _____

Proficiency Evaluation Form

Location _____ Student _____

Date _____ Evaluation Results | A   U |

Unusual Patient Characteristics _____

Time: Start _____ Stop _____ Total _____ (minutes)

Performance	Results	Comments
A. Check Order	A U N	
B. Review Chart	A U N	
C. Maintain Asepsis	A U N	
D. Obtain Equipment	A U N	
E. Assemble Equipment	A U N	
F. Test Equipment	A U N	
G. Confirm Patient	A U N	
H. Inform Patient	A U N	
I. Implement Procedure	A U N	
J. Monitor Patient	A U N	
K. Conclude Procedure	A U N	
L. Record Results	A U N	
M. Report Observations	A U N	

Additional Comments:

Signatures:

Student _____ Evaluator _____

Proficiency Evaluation Form

Location _____ Student _____

Date _____ Evaluation Results | A   U |

Unusual Patient Characteristics _____

Time: Start _____ Stop _____ Total _____ (minutes)

Performance	Results	Comments
A. Check Order	A U N	
B. Review Chart	A U N	
C. Maintain Asepsis	A U N	
D. Obtain Equipment	A U N	
E. Confirm Patient	A U N	
F. Inform Patient	A U N	
G. Implement Procedure	A U N	
H. Monitor Patient	A U N	
I. Conclude Procedure	A U N	
J. Record Results	A U N	
K. Report Observations	A U N	

Additional Comments:

Signatures:

Student _____ Evaluator _____

Proficiency Evaluation Form

Location _____ Student _____

Date _____ Evaluation Results | A   U |

Unusual Patient Characteristics _____

Time: Start _____ Stop _____ Total _____ (minutes)

Performance	Results	Comments
A. Maintain Asepsis	A U N	
B. Obtain Equipment	A U N	
C. Assemble Equipment	A U N	
D. Test Equipment	A U N	

Additional Comments:

Signatures:

Student _____ Evaluator _____

Proficiency Evaluation Form

Location _____ Student _____

Date _____ Evaluation Results | A   U |

Unusual Patient Characteristics _____

Time: Start _____ Stop _____ Total _____ (minutes)

Performance	Results	Comments
A. Maintain Asepsis	A U N	
B. Obtain Equipment	A U N	
C. Confirm Patient	A U N	
D. Inform Patient	A U N	
E. Implement Procedure	A U N	
F. Record Information	A U N	
G. Conclude Procedure	A U N	
H. Report Observations	A U N	

Additional Comments:

Signatures:

Student _____ Evaluator _____

Proficiency Evaluation Form

Location _____ Student _____

Date _____ Evaluation Results | A   U |

Unusual Patient Characteristics _____

Time: Start _____ Stop _____ Total _____ (minutes)

Performance	Results	Comments
A. Maintain Asepsis	A U N	
B. Obtain Equipment	A U N	
C. Confirm Patient	A U N	
D. Inform Patient	A U N	
E. Implement Procedure	A U N	
F. Conclude Procedure	A U N	
G. Report Observations	A U N	

Additional Comments:

Signatures:

Student _____ Evaluator _____

Proficiency Evaluation Form

Location _____ Student _____

Date _____ Evaluation Results | A   U |

Unusual Patient Characteristics _____

Time: Start _____ Stop _____ Total _____ (minutes)

Performance	Results	Comments
A. Check Order	A U N	
B. Review Chart	A U N	
C. Maintain Asepsis	A U N	
D. Obtain Equipment	A U N	
E. Confirm Patient	A U N	
F. Inform Patient	A U N	
G. Implement Procedure	A U N	
H. Conclude Procedure	A U N	
I. Report Observations	A U N	

Additional Comments:

Signatures:

Student _____ Evaluator _____

Proficiency Evaluation Form

Location _____   Student _____

Date _____   Evaluation Results | A   U |

Unusual Patient Characteristics _____

Time: Start _____ Stop _____ Total _____ (minutes)

Performance	Results	Comments
A. Check Order	A U N	
B. Review Chart	A U N	
C. Maintain Asepsis	A U N	
D. Obtain Equipment	A U N	
E. Assemble Equipment	A U N	
F. Test Equipment	A U N	
G. Confirm Patient	A U N	
H. Inform Patient	A U N	
I. Implement Procedure	A U N	
J. Conclude Procedure	A U N	
K. Report Observations	A U N	

Additional Comments:

Signatures:

Student _____ Evaluator _____

Proficiency Evaluation Form

Location _____ Student _____

Date _____ Evaluation Results | A   U |

Unusual Patient Characteristics _____

Time: Start _____ Stop _____ Total _____ (minutes)

Performance	Results	Comments
A. Check Order	A U N	
B. Review Chart	A U N	
C. Maintain Asepsis	A U N	
D. Obtain Equipment	A U N	
E. Assemble Equipment	A U N	
F. Test Equipment	A U N	
G. Confirm Patient	A U N	
H. Implement Patient	A U N	
I. Monitor Patient	A U N	
J. Record Results	A U N	
K. Report Observations	A U N	

Additional Comments:

Signatures:

Student _____ Evaluator _____

Proficiency Evaluation Form

Location _____ Student _____

Date _____ Evaluation Results | A   U |

Unusual Patient Characteristics _____

Time: Start _____ Stop _____ Total _____ (minutes)

Performance	Results	Comments
A. Maintain Asepsis	A U N	
B. Obtain Equipment	A U N	
C. Assemble Equipment	A U N	
D. Test Equipment	A U N	

Additional Comments:

Signatures:

Student _____ Evaluator _____

Proficiency Evaluation Form

Location _____ Student _____

Date _____ Evaluation Results | A   U |

Unusual Patient Characteristics _____

Time: Start _____ Stop _____ Total _____ (minutes)

Performance	Results	Comments
A. Maintain Asepsis	A U N	
B. Obtain Equipment	A U N	
C. Confirm Patient	A U N	
D. Implement Procedure	A U N	
E. Record Results	A U N	
F. Report Observations	A U N	

Additional Comments:

Signatures:

Student _____ Evaluator _____

Proficiency Evaluation Form

Location _____ Student _____

Date _____ Evaluation Results | A   U |

Unusual Patient Characteristics _____

Time: Start _____ Stop _____ Total _____ (minutes)

Performance	Results	Comments
A. Maintain Asepsis	A U N	
B. Obtain Equipment	A U N	
C. Confirm Patient	A U N	
D. Implement Procedure	A U N	
E. Report Observations	A U N	

Additional Comments:

Signatures:

Student _____ Evaluator _____

Appendix

Reprinted by the
U.S. DEPARTMENT OF HEALTH AND HUMAN SERVICES
PUBLIC HEALTH SERVICE
from MMWR, June 24, 1988, Vol. 37, No. 24, pp. 377-382, 387-388

Update: Universal Precautions for Prevention of Transmission of Human Immunodeficiency Virus, Hepatitis B Virus, and Other Bloodborne Pathogens in Health-Care Settings

Introduction

The purpose of this report is to clarify and supplement the CDC publication entitled "Recommendations for Prevention of HIV Transmission in Health-Care Settings" (1).*

In 1983, CDC published a document entitled "Guideline for Isolation Precautions in Hospitals" (2) that contained a section entitled "Blood and Body Fluid Precautions." The recommendations in this section called for blood and body fluid precautions when a patient was known or suspected to be infected with bloodborne pathogens. In August 1987, CDC published a document entitled "Recommendations for Prevention of HIV Transmission in Health-Care Settings" (1). In contrast to the 1983 document, the 1987 document recommended that blood and body fluid precautions be consistently used for all patients regardless of their bloodborne infection status. This extension of blood and body fluid precautions to **all** patients is referred to as "Universal Blood and Body Fluid Precautions" or "Universal Precautions." Under universal precautions, blood and certain body fluids of all patients are considered potentially infectious for human immunodeficiency virus (HIV), hepatitis B virus (HBV), and other bloodborne pathogens.

Universal precautions are intended to prevent parenteral, mucous membrane, and nonintact skin exposures of health-care workers to bloodborne pathogens. In addition, immunization with HBV vaccine is recommended as an important adjunct to universal precautions for health-care workers who have exposures to blood (3,4).

Since the recommendations for universal precautions were published in August 1987, CDC and the Food and Drug Administration (FDA) have received requests for clarification of the following issues: 1) body fluids to which universal precautions apply, 2) use of protective barriers, 3) use of gloves for phlebotomy, 4) selection of gloves for use while observing universal precautions, and 5) need for making changes in waste management programs as a result of adopting universal precautions.

---

*The August 1987 publication should be consulted for general information and specific recommendations not addressed in this update.

Copies of this report and of the *MMWR* supplement entitled *Recommendations for Prevention of HIV Transmission in Health-Care Settings* published in August 1987 are available through the National AIDS Information Clearinghouse, P.O. Box 6003, Rockville, MD 20850.

June 24, 1988;37:377-382, 387-388

Body Fluids to Which Universal Precautions Apply

Universal precautions apply to blood and to other body fluids containing visible blood. Occupational transmission of HIV and HBV to health-care workers by blood is documented (4,5). **Blood is the single most important source of HIV, HBV, and other bloodborne pathogens in the occupational setting. Infection control efforts for HIV, HBV, and other bloodborne pathogens must focus on preventing exposures to blood as well as on delivery of HBV immunization.**

Universal precautions also apply to semen and vaginal secretions. Although both of these fluids have been implicated in the sexual transmission of HIV and HBV, they have not been implicated in occupational transmission from patient to health-care worker. This observation is not unexpected, since exposure to semen in the usual health-care setting is limited, and the routine practice of wearing gloves for performing vaginal examinations protects health-care workers from exposure to potentially infectious vaginal secretions.

Universal precautions also apply to tissues and to the following fluids: cerebrospinal fluid (CSF), synovial fluid, pleural fluid, peritoneal fluid, pericardial fluid, and amniotic fluid. The risk of transmission of HIV and HBV from these fluids is unknown; epidemiologic studies in the health-care and community setting are currently inadequate to assess the potential risk to health-care workers from occupational exposures to them. However, HIV has been isolated from CSF, synovial, and amniotic fluid (6–8), and HBsAg has been detected in synovial fluid, amniotic fluid, and peritoneal fluid (9–11). One case of HIV transmission was reported after a percutaneous exposure to bloody pleural fluid obtained by needle aspiration (12). Whereas aseptic procedures used to obtain these fluids for diagnostic or therapeutic purposes protect health-care workers from skin exposures, they cannot prevent penetrating injuries due to contaminated needles or other sharp instruments.

Body Fluids to Which Universal Precautions Do Not Apply

Universal precautions do not apply to feces, nasal secretions, sputum, sweat, tears, urine, and vomitus unless they contain visible blood. The risk of transmission of HIV and HBV from these fluids and materials is extremely low or nonexistent. HIV has been isolated and HBsAg has been demonstrated in some of these fluids; however, epidemiologic studies in the health-care and community setting have not implicated these fluids or materials in the transmission of HIV and HBV infections (13,14). Some of the above fluids and excretions represent a potential source for nosocomial and community-acquired infections with other pathogens, and recommendations for preventing the transmission of nonbloodborne pathogens have been published (2).

Precautions for Other Body Fluids in Special Settings

Human breast milk has been implicated in perinatal transmission of HIV, and HBsAg has been found in the milk of mothers infected with HBV (10,13). However, occupational exposure to human breast milk has not been implicated in the transmission of HIV nor HBV infection to health-care workers. Moreover, the health-care worker will not have the same type of intensive exposure to breast milk as the nursing neonate. Whereas universal precautions do not apply to human breast milk, gloves may be worn by health-care workers in situations where exposures to breast milk might be frequent, for example, in breast milk banking.

Saliva of some persons infected with HBV has been shown to contain HBV-DNA at concentrations 1/1,000 to 1/10,000 of that found in the infected person's serum (15). HBsAg-positive saliva has been shown to be infectious when injected into experimental animals and in human bite exposures (16–18). However, HBsAg-positive saliva has not been shown to be infectious when applied to oral mucous membranes in experimental primate studies (18) or through contamination of musical instruments or cardiopulmonary resuscitation dummies used by HBV carriers (19,20). Epidemiologic studies of nonsexual household contacts of HIV-infected patients, including several small series in which HIV transmission failed to occur after bites or after percutaneous inoculation or contamination of cuts and open wounds with saliva from HIV-infected patients, suggest that the potential for salivary transmission of HIV is remote (5,13,14,21,22). One case report from Germany has suggested the possibility of transmission of HIV in a household setting from an infected child to a sibling through a human bite (23). The bite did not break the skin or result in bleeding. Since the date of seroconversion to HIV was not known for either child in this case, evidence for the role of saliva in the transmission of virus is unclear (23). Another case report suggested the possibility of transmission of HIV from husband to wife by contact with saliva during kissing (24). However, follow-up studies did not confirm HIV infection in the wife (21).

Universal precautions do not apply to saliva. General infection control practices already in existence — including the use of gloves for digital examination of mucous membranes and endotracheal suctioning, and handwashing after exposure to saliva — should further minimize the minute risk, if any, for salivary transmission of HIV and HBV (1,25). Gloves need not be worn when feeding patients and when wiping saliva from skin.

Special precautions, however, are recommended for dentistry (1). Occupationally acquired infection with HBV in dental workers has been documented (4), and two possible cases of occupationally acquired HIV infection involving dentists have been reported (5,26). During dental procedures, contamination of saliva with blood is predictable, trauma to health-care workers' hands is common, and blood spattering may occur. Infection control precautions for dentistry minimize the potential for nonintact skin and mucous membrane contact of dental health-care workers to blood-contaminated saliva of patients. In addition, the use of gloves for oral examinations and treatment in the dental setting may also protect the patient's oral mucous membranes from exposures to blood, which may occur from breaks in the skin of dental workers' hands.

Use of Protective Barriers

Protective barriers reduce the risk of exposure of the health-care worker's skin or mucous membranes to potentially infective materials. For universal precautions, protective barriers reduce the risk of exposure to blood, body fluids containing visible blood, and other fluids to which universal precautions apply. Examples of protective barriers include gloves, gowns, masks, and protective eyewear. Gloves should reduce the incidence of contamination of hands, but they cannot prevent penetrating injuries due to needles or other sharp instruments. Masks and protective eyewear or face shields should reduce the incidence of contamination of mucous membranes of the mouth, nose, and eyes.

June 24, 1988;37:377-382, 387-388

Universal precautions are intended to supplement rather than replace recommendations for routine infection control, such as handwashing and using gloves to prevent gross microbial contamination of hands (27). Because specifying the types of barriers needed for every possible clinical situation is impractical, some judgment must be exercised.

The risk of nosocomial transmission of HIV, HBV, and other bloodborne pathogens can be minimized if health-care workers use the following general guidelines:[†]

1. Take care to prevent injuries when using needles, scalpels, and other sharp instruments or devices; when handling sharp instruments after procedures; when cleaning used instruments; and when disposing of used needles. Do not recap used needles by hand; do not remove used needles from disposable syringes by hand; and do not bend, break, or otherwise manipulate used needles by hand. Place used disposable syringes and needles, scalpel blades, and other sharp items in puncture-resistant containers for disposal. Locate the puncture-resistant containers as close to the use area as is practical.

2. Use protective barriers to prevent exposure to blood, body fluids containing visible blood, and other fluids to which universal precautions apply. The type of protective barrier(s) should be appropriate for the procedure being performed and the type of exposure anticipated.

3. Immediately and thoroughly wash hands and other skin surfaces that are contaminated with blood, body fluids containing visible blood, or other body fluids to which universal precautions apply.

Glove Use for Phlebotomy

Gloves should reduce the incidence of blood contamination of hands during phlebotomy (drawing blood samples), but they cannot prevent penetrating injuries caused by needles or other sharp instruments. The likelihood of hand contamination with blood containing HIV, HBV, or other bloodborne pathogens during phlebotomy depends on several factors: 1) the skill and technique of the health-care worker, 2) the frequency with which the health-care worker performs the procedure (other factors being equal, the cumulative risk of blood exposure is higher for a health-care worker who performs more procedures), 3) whether the procedure occurs in a routine or emergency situation (where blood contact may be more likely), and 4) the prevalence of infection with bloodborne pathogens in the patient population. The likelihood of infection after skin exposure to blood containing HIV or HBV will depend on the concentration of virus (viral concentration is much higher for hepatitis B than for HIV), the duration of contact, the presence of skin lesions on the hands of the health-care worker, and — for HBV — the immune status of the health-care worker. Although not accurately quantified, the risk of HIV infection following intact skin contact with infective blood is certainly much less than the 0.5% risk following percutaneous needlestick exposures (5). In universal precautions, *all* blood is assumed to be potentially infective for bloodborne pathogens, but in certain settings (e.g., volunteer blood-donation centers) the prevalence of infection with some bloodborne pathogens (e.g., HIV, HBV) is known to be very low. Some institutions have relaxed recommendations for using gloves for phlebotomy procedures by skilled phlebotomists in settings where the prevalence of bloodborne pathogens is known to be very low.

[†]The August 1987 publication should be consulted for general information and specific recommendations not addressed in this update.

June 24, 1988;37:377-382, 387-388

Institutions that judge that routine gloving for *all* phlebotomies is not necessary should periodically reevaluate their policy. Gloves should always be available to health-care workers who wish to use them for phlebotomy. In addition, the following general guidelines apply:

1. Use gloves for performing phlebotomy when the health-care worker has cuts, scratches, or other breaks in his/her skin.
2. Use gloves in situations where the health-care worker judges that hand contamination with blood may occur, for example, when performing phlebotomy on an uncooperative patient.
3. Use gloves for performing finger and/or heel sticks on infants and children.
4. Use gloves when persons are receiving training in phlebotomy.

Selection of Gloves

The Center for Devices and Radiological Health, FDA, has responsibility for regulating the medical glove industry. Medical gloves include those marketed as sterile surgical or nonsterile examination gloves made of vinyl or latex. General purpose utility ("rubber") gloves are also used in the health-care setting, but they are not regulated by FDA since they are not promoted for medical use. There are no reported differences in barrier effectiveness between intact latex and intact vinyl used to manufacture gloves. Thus, the type of gloves selected should be appropriate for the task being performed.

The following general guidelines are recommended:

1. Use sterile gloves for procedures involving contact with normally sterile areas of the body.
2. Use examination gloves for procedures involving contact with mucous membranes, unless otherwise indicated, and for other patient care or diagnostic procedures that do not require the use of sterile gloves.
3. Change gloves between patient contacts.
4. Do not wash or disinfect surgical or examination gloves for reuse. Washing with surfactants may cause "wicking," i.e., the enhanced penetration of liquids through undetected holes in the glove. Disinfecting agents may cause deterioration.
5. Use general-purpose utility gloves (e.g., rubber household gloves) for housekeeping chores involving potential blood contact and for instrument cleaning and decontamination procedures. Utility gloves may be decontaminated and reused but should be discarded if they are peeling, cracked, or discolored, or if they have punctures, tears, or other evidence of deterioration.

Waste Management

Universal precautions are not intended to change waste management programs previously recommended by CDC for health-care settings (*1*). Policies for defining, collecting, storing, decontaminating, and disposing of infective waste are generally determined by institutions in accordance with state and local regulations. Information regarding waste management regulations in health-care settings may be obtained from state or local health departments or agencies responsible for waste management.

Reported by: Center for Devices and Radiological Health, Food and Drug Administration. Hospital Infections Program, AIDS Program, and Hepatitis Br, Div of Viral Diseases, Center for Infectious Diseases, National Institute for Occupational Safety and Health, CDC.

June 24, 1988;37:377-382, 387-388

Editorial Note: Implementation of universal precautions does not eliminate the need for other category- or disease-specific isolation precautions, such as enteric precautions for infectious diarrhea or isolation for pulmonary tuberculosis (*1,2*). In addition to universal precautions, detailed precautions have been developed for the following procedures and/or settings in which prolonged or intensive exposures to blood occur: invasive procedures, dentistry, autopsies or morticians' services, dialysis, and the clinical laboratory. These detailed precautions are found in the August 21, 1987, "Recommendations for Prevention of HIV Transmission in Health-Care Settings" (*1*). In addition, specific precautions have been developed for research laboratories (*28*).

References

1. Centers for Disease Control. Recommendations for prevention of HIV transmission in health-care settings. MMWR 1987;36(suppl no. 2S).
2. Garner JS, Simmons BP. Guideline for isolation precautions in hospitals. Infect Control 1983:4;245–325.
3. Immunization Practices Advisory Committee. Recommendations for protection against viral hepatitis. MMWR 1985;34:313-24,329–35.
4. Department of Labor, Department of Health and Human Services. Joint advisory notice: protection against occupational exposure to hepatitis B virus (HBV) and human immuno-deficiency virus (HIV). Washington, DC:US Department of Labor, US Department of Health and Human Services, 1987.
5. Centers for Disease Control. Update: Acquired immunodeficiency syndrome and human immunodeficiency virus infection among health-care workers. MMWR 1988;37:229–34,239.
6. Hollander H, Levy JA. Neurologic abnormalities and recovery of human immunodeficiency virus from cerebrospinal fluid. Ann Intern Med 1987;106:692–5.
7. Wirthrington RH, Cornes P, Harris JRW, et al. Isolation of human immunodeficiency virus from synovial fluid of a patient with reactive arthritis. Br Med J 1987;294:484.
8. Mundy DC, Schinazi RF, Gerber AR, Nahmias AJ, Randall HW. Human immunodeficiency virus isolated from amniotic fluid. Lancet 1987;2:459–60.
9. Onion DK, Crumpacker CS, Gilliland BC. Arthritis of hepatitis associated with Australia antigen. Ann Intern Med 1971;75:29–33.
10. Lee AKY, Ip HMH, Wong VCW. Mechanisms of maternal-fetal transmission of hepatitis B virus. J Infect Dis 1978;138:668–71.
11. Bond WW, Petersen NJ, Gravelle CR, Favero MS. Hepatitis B virus in peritoneal dialysis fluid: A potential hazard. Dialysis and Transplantation 1982;11:592–600.
12. Oskenhendler E, Harzic M, Le Roux J-M, Rabian C, Clauvel JP. HIV infection with serocon-version after a superficial needlestick injury to the finger [Letter]. N Engl J Med 1986;315:582.
13. Lifson AR. Do alternate modes for transmission of human immunodeficiency virus exist? A review. JAMA 1988;259:1353–6.
14. Friedland GH, Saltzman BR, Rogers MF, et al. Lack of transmission of HTLV-III/LAV infection to household contacts of patients with AIDS or AIDS-related complex with oral candidiasis. N Engl J Med 1986;314:344–9.
15. Jenison SA, Lemon SM, Baker LN, Newbold JE. Quantitative analysis of hepatitis B virus DNA in saliva and semen of chronically infected homosexual men. J Infect Dis 1987;156:299–306.
16. Cancio-Bello TP, de Medina M, Shorey J, Valledor MD, Schiff ER. An institutional outbreak of hepatitis B related to a human biting carrier. J Infect Dis 1982;146:652–6.
17. MacQuarrie MB, Forghani B, Wolochow DA. Hepatitis B transmitted by a human bite. JAMA 1974;230:723–4.
18. Scott RM, Snitbhan R, Bancroft WH, Alter HJ, Tingpalapong M. Experimental transmission of hepatitis B virus by semen and saliva. J Infect Dis 1980;142:67–71.

19. Glaser JB, Nadler JP. Hepatitis B virus in a cardiopulmonary resuscitation training course: Risk of transmission from a surface antigen-positive participant. Arch Intern Med 1985;145:1653–5.
20. Osterholm MT, Bravo ER, Crosson JT, et al. Lack of transmission of viral hepatitis type B after oral exposure to HBsAg-positive saliva. Br Med J 1979;2:1263–4.
21. Curran JW, Jaffe HW, Hardy AM, et al. Epidemiology of HIV infection and AIDS in the United States. Science 1988;239:610–6.
22. Jason JM, McDougal JS, Dixon G, et al. HTLV-III/LAV antibody and immune status of household contacts and sexual partners of persons with hemophilia. JAMA 1986;255:212–5.
23. Wahn V, Kramer HH, Voit T, Brüster HT, Scrampical B, Scheid A. Horizontal transmission of HIV infection between two siblings [Letter]. Lancet 1986;2:694.
24. Salahuddin SZ, Groopman JE, Markham PD, et al. HTLV-III in symptom-free seronegative persons. Lancet 1984;2:1418–20.
25. Simmons BP, Wong ES. Guideline for prevention of nosocomial pneumonia. Atlanta: US Department of Health and Human Services, Public Health Service, Centers for Disease Control, 1982.
26. Klein RS, Phelan JA, Freeman K, et al. Low occupational risk of human immunodeficiency virus infection among dental professionals. N Engl J Med 1988;318:86–90.
27. Garner JS, Favero MS. Guideline for handwashing and hospital environmental control, 1985. Atlanta: US Department of Health and Human Services, Public Health Service, Centers for Disease Control, 1985; HHS publication no. 99-1117.
28. Centers for Disease Control. 1988 Agent summary statement for human immunodeficiency virus and report on laboratory-acquired infection with human immunodeficiency virus. MMWR 1988;37(suppl no. S4:1S-22S).

☆U.S. GOVERNMENT PRINTING OFFICE: 1988-530-009/84718

REPRINTED BY
U.S. DEPARTMENT OF HEALTH AND HUMAN SERVICES
PUBLIC HEALTH SERVICE
FROM THE
MORBIDITY AND MORTALITY WEEKLY REPORT
RECOMMENDATIONS AND REPORTS
July 12, 1991 / Vol. 40 / No. RR-8
Pages 1-9

Recommendations for Preventing Transmission of Human Immunodeficiency Virus and Hepatitis B Virus to Patients During Exposure-Prone Invasive Procedures

U.S. DEPARTMENT OF HEALTH AND HUMAN SERVICES
Public Health Service
Centers for Disease Control
Atlanta, Georgia 30333

Recommendations for Preventing Transmission of Human Immunodeficiency Virus and Hepatitis B Virus to Patients During Exposure-Prone Invasive Procedures

This document has been developed by the Centers for Disease Control (CDC) to update recommendations for prevention of transmission of human immunodeficiency virus (HIV) and hepatitis B virus (HBV) in the health-care setting. Current data suggest that the risk for such transmission from a health-care worker (HCW) to a patient during an invasive procedure is small; a precise assessment of the risk is not yet available. This document contains recommendations to provide guidance for prevention of HIV and HBV transmission during those invasive procedures that are considered exposure-prone.

INTRODUCTION

Recommendations have been made by the Centers for Disease Control (CDC) for the prevention of transmission of the human immunodeficiency virus (HIV) and the hepatitis B virus (HBV) in health-care settings (1-6). These recommendations emphasize adherence to universal precautions that require that blood and other specified body fluids of **all** patients be handled as if they contain blood-borne pathogens (1,2).

Previous guidelines contained precautions to be used during invasive procedures (defined in Appendix) and recommendations for the management of HIV- and HBV-infected health-care workers (HCWs) (1). These guidelines did not include specific recommendations on testing HCWs for HIV or HBV infection, and they did not provide guidance on which invasive procedures may represent increased risk to the patient.

The recommendations outlined in this document are based on the following considerations:

- Infected HCWs who adhere to universal precautions and who do not perform invasive procedures pose no risk for transmitting HIV or HBV to patients.

- Infected HCWs who adhere to universal precautions and who perform certain exposure-prone procedures (see page 4) pose a small risk for transmitting HBV to patients.

- HIV is transmitted much less readily than HBV.

In the interim, until further data are available, additional precautions are prudent to prevent HIV and HBV transmission during procedures that have been linked to HCW-to-patient HBV transmission or that are considered exposure-prone.

BACKGROUND

Infection-Control Practices

Previous recommendations have specified that infection-control programs should incorporate principles of universal precautions (i.e., appropriate use of hand washing, protective barriers, and care in the use and disposal of needles and other sharp instruments) and should maintain these precautions rigorously in all health-care settings (1,2,5). Proper application of these principles will assist in minimizing the risk of transmission of HIV or HBV from patient to HCW, HCW to patient, or patient to patient.

1

As part of standard infection-control practice, instruments and other reusable equipment used in performing invasive procedures should be appropriately disinfected and sterilized as follows (7):

- Equipment and devices that enter the patient's vascular system or other normally sterile areas of the body should be sterilized before being used for each patient.
- Equipment and devices that touch intact mucous membranes but do not penetrate the patient's body surfaces should be sterilized when possible or undergo high-level disinfection if they cannot be sterilized before being used for each patient.
- Equipment and devices that do not touch the patient or that only touch intact skin of the patient need only be cleaned with a detergent or as indicated by the manufacturer.

Compliance with universal precautions and recommendations for disinfection and sterilization of medical devices should be scrupulously monitored in all health-care settings (1, 7, 8). Training of HCWs in proper infection-control technique should begin in professional and vocational schools and continue as an ongoing process. Institutions should provide all HCWs with appropriate inservice education regarding infection control and safety and should establish procedures for monitoring compliance with infection-control policies.

All HCWs who might be exposed to blood in an occupational setting should receive hepatitis B vaccine, preferably during their period of professional training and before any occupational exposures could occur (8, 9).

Transmission of HBV During Invasive Procedures

Since the introduction of serologic testing for HBV infection in the early 1970s, there have been published reports of 20 clusters in which a total of over 300 patients were infected with HBV in association with treatment by an HBV-infected HCW. In 12 of these clusters, the implicated HCW did not routinely wear gloves; several HCWs also had skin lesions that may have facilitated HBV transmission (10-22). These 12 clusters included nine linked to dentists or oral surgeons and one cluster each linked to a general practitioner, an inhalation therapist, and a cardiopulmonary-bypass-pump technician. The clusters associated with the inhalation therapist and the cardiopulmonary-bypass-pump technician — and some of the other 10 clusters — could possibly have been prevented if current recommendations on universal precautions, including glove use, had been in effect. In the remaining eight clusters, transmission occurred despite glove use by the HCWs; five clusters were linked to obstetricians or gynecologists, and three were linked to cardiovascular surgeons (6, 22-28). In addition, recent unpublished reports strongly suggest HBV transmission from three surgeons to patients in 1989 and 1990 during colorectal (CDC, unpublished data), abdominal, and cardiothoracic surgery (29).

Seven of the HCWs who were linked to published clusters in the United States were allowed to perform invasive procedures following modification of invasive techniques (e.g., double gloving and restriction of certain high-risk procedures) (6,11- 13,15,16, 24). For five HCWs, no further transmission to patients was observed. In two instances involving an obstetrician/gynecologist and an oral surgeon, HBV was transmitted to patients after techniques were modified (6, 12).

Review of the 20 published studies indicates that a combination of risk factors accounted for transmission of HBV from HCWs to patients. Of the HCWs whose hepatitis B e antigen (HBeAg) status was determined (17 of 20), all were HBeAg positive. The presence of HBeAg in serum is associated with higher levels of circulating virus and therefore with greater infectivity of hepatitis-B-surface-antigen (HBsAg)-positive individuals; the risk of HBV transmission to an HCW after a percutaneous exposure to HBeAg-positive blood is approximately 30% (30-32). In addition, each report indicated that the potential existed for contamination of surgical wounds or traumatized tissue, either from a major break in standard infection-control practices (e.g., not wearing gloves during invasive procedures) or from unintentional injury to the infected HCW during invasive procedures (e.g., needle sticks incurred while manipulating needles without being able to see them during suturing).

Most reported clusters in the United States occurred before awareness increased of the risks of transmission of blood-borne pathogens in health-care settings and before emphasis was placed on the use of universal precautions and hepatitis B vaccine among HCWs. The limited number of reports of HBV transmission from HCWs to patients in recent years may reflect the adoption of universal precautions and increased use of HBV vaccine. However, the limited number of recent reports does not preclude the occurrence of undetected or unreported small clusters or individual instances of transmission; routine use of gloves does not prevent most injuries caused by sharp instruments and does not eliminate the potential for exposure of a patient to an HCW's blood and transmission of HBV (*6, 22-29*).

Transmission of HIV During Invasive Procedures

The risk of HIV transmission to an HCW after percutaneous exposure to HIV-infected blood is considerably lower than the risk of HBV transmission after percutaneous exposure to HBeAg-positive blood (0.3% versus approximately 30%) (*33-35*). Thus, the risk of transmission of HIV from an infected HCW to a patient during an invasive procedure is likely to be proportionately lower than the risk of HBV transmission from an HBeAg-positive HCW to a patient during the same procedure. As with HBV, the relative infectivity of HIV probably varies among individuals and over time for a single individual. Unlike HBV infection, however, there is currently no readily available laboratory test for increased HIV infectivity.

Investigation of a cluster of HIV infections among patients in the practice of one dentist with acquired immunodeficiency syndrome (AIDS) strongly suggested that HIV was transmitted to five of the approximately 850 patients evaluated through June 1991 (*36-38*). The investigation indicates that HIV transmission occurred during dental care, although the precise mechanisms of transmission have not been determined. In two other studies, when patients cared for by a general surgeon and a surgical resident who had AIDS were tested, all patients tested, 75 and 62, respectively, were negative for HIV infection (*39, 40*). In a fourth study, 143 patients who had been treated by a dental student with HIV infection and were later tested were all negative for HIV infection (*41*). In another investigation, HIV antibody testing was offered to all patients whose surgical procedures had been performed by a general surgeon within 7 years before the surgeon's diagnosis of AIDS; the date at which the surgeon became infected with HIV is unknown (*42*). Of 1,340 surgical patients contacted, 616 (46%) were tested for HIV. One patient, a known intravenous drug user, was HIV positive when tested but may already have been infected at the time of surgery. HIV test results for the 615 other surgical patients were negative (95% confidence interval for risk of transmission per operation = 0.0%-0.5%).

The limited number of participants and the differences in procedures associated with these five investigations limit the ability to generalize from them and to define precisely the risk of HIV transmission from HIV-infected HCWs to patients. A precise estimate of the risk of HIV transmission from infected HCWs to patients can be determined only after careful evaluation of a substantially larger number of patients whose exposure-prone procedures have been performed by HIV-infected HCWs.

Exposure-Prone Procedures

Despite adherence to the principles of universal precautions, certain invasive surgical and dental procedures have been implicated in the transmission of HBV from infected HCWs to patients, and should be considered exposure-prone. Reported examples include certain oral, cardiothoracic, colorectal (CDC, unpublished data), and obstetric/gynecologic procedures (*6, 12, 22-29*).

Certain other invasive procedures should also be considered exposure-prone. In a prospective study CDC conducted in four hospitals, one or more percutaneous injuries occurred among surgical personnel during 96 (6.9%) of 1,382 operative procedures on the general surgery, gynecology, orthopedic, cardiac, and trauma services (*43*). Percutaneous exposure of the patient to the HCW's blood may have occurred when the sharp object causing the injury recontacted the patient's open wound in 28 (32%) of the 88 observed injuries to surgeons (range among surgical specialties = 8%-57%; range among hospitals = 24%-42%).

> **Characteristics of exposure-prone procedures include digital palpation of a needle tip in a body cavity or the simultaneous presence of the HCW's fingers and a needle or other sharp instrument or object in a poorly visualized or highly confined anatomic site. Performance of exposure-prone procedures presents a recognized risk of percutaneous injury to the HCW, and — if such an injury occurs — the HCW's blood is likely to contact the patient's body cavity, subcutaneous tissues, and/or mucous membranes.**

Experience with HBV indicates that invasive procedures that do not have the above characteristics would be expected to pose substantially lower risk, if any, of transmission of HIV and other blood-borne pathogens from an infected HCW to patients.

RECOMMENDATIONS

Investigations of HIV and HBV transmission from HCWs to patients indicate that, when HCWs adhere to recommended infection-control procedures, the risk of transmitting HBV from an infected HCW to a patient is small, and the risk of transmitting HIV is likely to be even smaller. However, the likelihood of exposure of the patient to an HCW's blood is greater for certain procedures designated as exposure-prone. To minimize the risk of HIV or HBV transmission, the following measures are recommended:

- **All HCWs should adhere to universal precautions, including the appropriate use of hand washing, protective barriers, and care in the use and disposal of needles and other sharp instruments. HCWs who have exudative lesions or weeping dermatitis should refrain from all direct patient care and from handling patient-care equipment and devices used in performing invasive procedures until the condition resolves. HCWs should also comply with current guidelines for disinfection and sterilization of reusable devices used in invasive procedures.**

- **Currently available data provide no basis for recommendations to restrict the practice of HCWs infected with HIV or HBV who perform invasive procedures not identified as exposure-prone, provided the infected HCWs practice recommended surgical or dental technique and comply with universal precautions and current recommendations for sterilization/disinfection.**

- **Exposure-prone procedures should be identified by medical/surgical/dental organizations and institutions at which the procedures are performed.**

- **HCWs who perform exposure-prone procedures should know their HIV antibody status. HCWs who perform exposure-prone procedures and who do not have serologic evidence of immunity to HBV from vaccination or from previous infection should know their HBsAg status and, if that is positive, should also know their HBeAg status.**

- **HCWs who are infected with HIV or HBV (and are HBeAg positive) should not perform exposure-prone procedures unless they have sought counsel from an expert review panel and been advised under what circumstances, if any, they may continue to perform these procedures.* Such circumstances would include notifying prospective patients of the HCW's seropositivity before they undergo exposure-prone invasive procedures.**

- **Mandatory testing of HCWs for HIV antibody, HBsAg, or HBeAg is not recommended. The current assessment of the risk that infected HCWs will transmit HIV or HBV to patients during exposure-prone procedures does not support the diversion of resources that would be required to implement mandatory testing programs. Compliance by HCWs with recommendations can be increased through education, training, and appropriate confidentiality safeguards.**

HCWS WHOSE PRACTICES ARE MODIFIED BECAUSE OF HIV OR HBV STATUS

HCWs whose practices are modified because of their HIV or HBV infection status should, whenever possible, be provided opportunities to continue appropriate patient-care activities. Career counseling and job retraining should be encouraged to promote the continued use of the HCW's talents, knowledge, and skills. HCWs whose practices are modified because of HBV infection should be reevaluated periodically to determine whether their HBeAg status changes due to resolution of infection or as a result of treatment (44).

---

*The review panel should include experts who represent a balanced perspective. Such experts might include all of the following: a) the HCW's personal physician(s), b) an infectious disease specialist with expertise in the epidemiology of HIV and HBV transmission, c) a health professional with expertise in the procedures performed by the HCW, and d) state or local public health official(s). If the HCW's practice is institutionally based, the expert review panel might also include a member of the infection-control committee, preferably a hospital epidemiologist. HCWs who perform exposure-prone procedures outside the hospital/institutional setting should seek advice from appropriate state and local public health officials regarding the review process. Panels must recognize the importance of confidentiality and the privacy rights of infected HCWs.

NOTIFICATION OF PATIENTS AND FOLLOW-UP STUDIES

The public health benefit of notification of patients who have had exposure-prone procedures performed by HCWs infected with HIV or positive for HBeAg should be considered on a case-by-case basis, taking into consideration an assessment of specific risks, confidentiality issues, and available resources. Carefully designed and implemented follow-up studies are necessary to determine more precisely the risk of transmission during such procedures. Decisions regarding notification and follow-up studies should be made in consultation with state and local public health officials.

ADDITIONAL NEEDS

- Clearer definition of the nature, frequency, and circumstances of blood contact between patients and HCWs during invasive procedures.

- Development and evaluation of new devices, protective barriers, and techniques that may prevent such blood contact without adversely affecting the quality of patient care.

- More information on the potential for HIV and HBV transmission through contaminated instruments.

- Improvements in sterilization and disinfection techniques for certain reusable equipment and devices.

- Identification of factors that may influence the likelihood of HIV or HBV transmission after exposure to HIV- or HBV-infected blood.

References
1. CDC. Recommendations for prevention of HIV transmission in health-care settings. MMWR 1987;36(suppl. no. 2S):1-18S.
2. CDC. Update: Universal precautions for prevention of transmission of human immunodeficiency virus, hepatitis B virus, and other bloodborne pathogens in health-care settings. MMWR 1988;37:377-82,387-8.
3. CDC. Hepatitis Surveillance Report No. 48. Atlanta: U.S. Department of Health and Human Services, Public Health Service, 1982:2-3.
4. CDC. CDC Guideline for Infection Control in Hospital Personnel, Atlanta, Georgia: Public Health Service, 1983. 24 pages. (GPO# 6AR031488305).
5. CDC. Guidelines for prevention of transmission of human immunodeficiency virus and hepatitis B virus to health-care and public-safety workers. MMWR 1989;38;(suppl. no. S-6):1-37.
6. Lettau LA, Smith JD, Williams D, et al. Transmission of hepatitis B with resultant restriction of surgical practice. JAMA 1986;255:934-7.
7. CDC. Guidelines for the prevention and control of nosocomial infections: guideline for handwashing and hospital environmental control. Atlanta, Georgia: Public Health Service, 1985. 20 pages. (GPO# 544-436/24441).
8. Department of Labor, Occupational Safety and Health Administration. Occupational exposure to bloodborne pathogens: proposed rule and notice of hearing. Federal Register 1989;54:23042-139.
9. CDC. Protection against viral hepatitis: recommendations of the immunization practices advisory committee (ACIP). MMWR 1990;39;(no. RR-2).
10. Levin ML, Maddrey WC, Wands JR, Mendeloff AI. Hepatitis B transmission by dentists. JAMA 1974;228:1139-40.
11. Rimland D, Parkin WE, Miller GB, Schrack WD. Hepatitis B outbreak traced to an oral surgeon. N Engl J Med 1977;296:953-8.
12. Goodwin D, Fannin SL, McCracken BB. An oral-surgeon related hepatitis-B outbreak. California Morbidity 1976;14.
13. Hadler SC, Sorley DL, Acree KH, et al. An outbreak of hepatitis B in a dental practice. Ann Intern Med 1981;95:133-8.
14. Reingold AL, Kane MA, Murphy BL, Checko P, Francis DP, Maynard JE. Transmission of hepatitis B by an oral surgeon. J Infect Dis 1982;145:262-8.
15. Goodman RA, Ahtone JL, Finton RJ. Hepatitis B transmission from dental personnel to patients: unfinished business [Editorial]. Ann Intern Med 1982;96:119.
16. Ahtone J, Goodman RA. Hepatitis B and dental personnel: transmission to patients and prevention issues. J Am Dent Assoc 1983;106:219-22.
17. Shaw FE, Jr, Barrett CL, Hamm R, et al. Lethal outbreak of hepatitis B in a dental practice. JAMA 1986;255:3260-4.
18. CDC. Outbreak of hepatitis B associated with an oral surgeon, New Hampshire. MMWR 1987;36:132-3.
19. Grob PJ, Moeschlin P. Risk to contacts of a medical practitioner carrying HBsAg. [Letter]. N Engl J Med 1975;293:197.
20. Grob PJ, Bischof B, Naeff F. Cluster of hepatitis B transmitted by a physician. Lancet 1981;2:1218-20.
21. Snydman DR, Hindman SH, Wineland MD, Bryan JA, Maynard JE. Nosocomial viral hepatitis B. A cluster among staff with subsequent transmission to patients. Ann Intern Med 1976;85:573-7.
22. Coutinho RA, Albrecht-van Lent P, Stoutjesdijk L, et al. Hepatitis B from doctors [Letter]. Lancet 1982;1:345-6.
23. Anonymous. Acute hepatitis B associated with gynaecological surgery. Lancet 1980;1:1-6.

24. Carl M, Blakey DL, Francis DP, Maynard JE. Interruption of hepatitis B transmission by modification of a gynaecologist's surgical technique. Lancet 1982;1:731-3.
25. Anonymous. Acute hepatitis B following gynaecological surgery. J Hosp Infect 1987;9:34-8.
26. Welch J, Webster M, Tilzey AJ, Noah ND, Banatvala JE. Hepatitis B infections after gynaecological surgery. Lancet 1989;1:205-7.
27. Haeram JW, Siebke JC, Ulstrup J, Geiram D, Helle I. HBsAg transmission from a cardiac surgeon incubating hepatitis B resulting in chronic antigenemia in four patients. Acta Med Scand 1981;210:389-92.
28. Flower AJE, Prentice M, Morgan G, et al. Hepatitis B infection following cardiothoracic surgery [Abstract]. 1990 International Symposium on Viral Hepatitis and Liver Diseases, Houston. 1990;94.
29. Heptonstall J. Outbreaks of hepatitis B virus infection associated with infected surgical staff in the United Kingdom. Communicable Disease Reports 1991 (in press).
30. Alter HJ, Seef LB, Kaplan PM, et al. Type B hepatitis: the infectivity of blood positive for e antigen and DNA polymerase after accidental needlestick exposure. N Engl J Med 1976;295:909-13.
31. Seeff LB, Wright EC, Zimmerman HJ, et al. Type B hepatitis after needlestick exposure: prevention with hepatitis B immunoglobulin: final report of the Veterans Administration Cooperative Study. Ann Intern Med 1978;88:285-93.
32. Grady GF, Lee VA, Prince AM, et al. Hepatitis B immune globulin for accidental exposures among medical personnel: final report of a multicenter controlled trial. J Infect Dis 1978;138:625-38.
33. Henderson DK, Fahey BJ, Willy M, et al. Risk for occupational transmission of human immunodeficiency virus type 1 (HIV-1) associated with clinical exposures: a prospective evaluation. Ann Intern Med 1990;113:740-6.
34. Marcus R, CDC Cooperative Needlestick Study Group. Surveillance of health-care workers exposed to blood from patients infected with the human immunodeficiency virus. N Engl J Med 1988;319:1118-23.
35. Gerberding JL, Bryant-LeBlanc CE, Nelson K, et al. Risk of transmitting the human immunodeficiency virus, cytomegalovirus, and hepatitis B virus to health-care workers exposed to patients with AIDS and AIDS-related conditions. J Infect Dis 1987;156:1-8.
36. CDC. Possible transmission of human immunodeficiency virus to a patient during an invasive dental procedure. MMWR 1990;39:489-93.
37. CDC. Update: transmission of HIV infection during an invasive dental procedure - Florida. MMWR 1991; 40:21-27,33.
38. CDC. Update: transmission of HIV infection during invasive dental procedures - Florida. MMWR 1991; 40:377-81.
39. Porter JD, Cruikshank JG, Gentle PH, Robinson RG, Gill ON. Management of patients treated by a surgeon with HIV infection. [Letter] Lancet 1990;335:113-4.
40. Armstrong FP, Miner JC, Wolfe WH. Investigation of a health-care worker with symptomatic human immunodeficiency virus infection: an epidemiologic approach. Milit Med 1987;152:414-8.
41. Comer RW, Myers DR, Steadman CD, Carter MJ, Rissing JP, Tedesco FJ. Management considerations for an HIV positive dental student. J Dent Educ 1991;55:187-91.
42. Mishu B, Schaffner W, Horan JM, Wood LH, Hutcheson R, McNabb P. A surgeon with AIDS: lack of evidence of transmission to patients. JAMA 1990;264:467-70.
43. Tokars J, Bell D, Marcus R, et al. Percutaneous injuries during surgical procedures [Abstract]. VII International Conference on AIDS. Vol 2. Florence, Italy, June 16-21, 1991:83.
44. Perrillo RP, Schiff ER, Davis GL, et al. A randomized, controlled trial of interferon alfa-2b alone and after prednisone withdrawal for the treatment of chronic hepatitis B. N Engl J Med 1990;323:295-301.

APPENDIX

Definition of Invasive Procedure

An invasive procedure is defined as "surgical entry into tissues, cavities, or organs or repair of major traumatic injuries" associated with any of the following: "1) an operating or delivery room, emergency department, or outpatient setting, including both physicians' and dentists' offices; 2) cardiac catheterization and angiographic procedures; 3) a vaginal or cesarean delivery or other invasive obstetric procedure during which bleeding may occur; or 4) the manipulation, cutting, or removal of any oral or perioral tissues, including tooth structure, during which bleeding occurs or the potential for bleeding exists."

Reprinted from: Centers for Disease Control. Recommendation for prevention of HIV transmission in health-care settings. *MMWR* 1987;36 (suppl. no. 2S):6S-7S.

PM72B3651079120

7

*U.S. Government Printing Office: 1991 — 531-011/42579